Intense Transformation

Discover How HIIT—the Most
Powerful Exercise to Transform
Your Mind, Body, & Spirit—Can
Activate Your Full Potential

Paul W. Matthews

within this book has been derived from various sources. Please consult a licensed professional before attempting any techniques outlined in this book.

By reading this document, the reader agrees that under no circumstances is the author responsible for any losses, direct or indirect, that are incurred as a result of the use of the information contained within this document, including, but not limited to, errors, omissions, or inaccuracies.

Table of Contents

Preface

High intensity interval training, known as HIIT, is a timeless method of body conditioning and training. Utilized by civilizations as early as the ancient Greeks all the way through the military might of the Roman Empire and through today. Unlike other "fad" exercises, the staying power of HIIT is reinforced by both its effectiveness and simplicity. By doing HIIT, you push the limits and boundaries of yourself as an individual, and the mind, body and spirit as a whole. You can achieve profound transformation simply by committing to HIIT. This is the be-all and end-all for no other exercise has come close to matching it in terms of power, strength, and intensity. Allow yourself to harness the power of high intensity interval training, may it transform your entire being.

Introduction

The History of High-Intensity Interval Training (HIIT)

Ancient Origins of Interval Training

You could be forgiven for thinking that high-intensity interval training is a 'modern' invention. It's everywhere: in gym classes, on YouTube, fitness apps, and there are countless companies which push to sell 'HIIT packages' as part of exorbitantly-priced 'deals.' The world we live in today is so full of fleeting fitness fads that it's easy to forget when something sticks around and just becomes a part of the cultural norm. HIIT is one of those cultural norms. It's available to everyone through various means, and anyone can do it.

The history of interval training is really quite interesting and stretches back further than you might think. If you were to step into a time machine and travel back to ancient Greece to meet the earliest Olympic athletes, what would you see? Who would you meet first? How do you think they might train? You might meet Milo of Croton in the middle of bench-pressing a fully grown bull, or you might wander down to the local palaestra where you will find some very buff men discussing the latest in philosophy.

At the time of writing this book, information regarding this is limited. However, the accounts which do exist help us create a broader understanding of the history of athletics. High-intensity interval training, before we came to know it as such, existed in one form or another, by many different names. The early Olympic athletes would have trained in a specialty gym known as a "xystos," and they were trained by former Olympic champions.

What about the training? How did the former champions train their charges? As far as we know, rigorously. Full-time training was not always available, although we do know that students used a mixture of bodyweight exercises and aerobic training to help strengthen their bodies. Athletes would have to train at home if they couldn't make the time to train at the xystos. This is where the bulk of bodyweight training would happen, and body conditioning would happen in the form of longform interval running exercises.

We also know that the ancient Olympic athletes trained according to their sport. Runners would run long distances, and fighters would focus on upper body strength.

In order to excel, athletes kept to a rigid four-day schedule known as a tetrad, which would look something like this (Britanniae, 2017):

Day One: Preparatory exercises

Day Two: Intense strength training

Day Three: Rest

Day Four: Moderate intensity training

Their training would continue following this pattern. Results could vary depending on the sport. Runners, for example, would have incredibly strong legs but no upper body strength, while fighters would be broad in the chest but narrow in the lower body.

Galenus, an ancient Greek doctor, was heavily critical of this level of athletic training. Most notably, he wanted there to be more substance to the training. He claimed that athletes were spending too much time focusing on their physical talents rather than their rational talents.

What can we, in the modern era, take from this? Galenus makes a solid case for training the mind as well as the body. Athletes were often so drawn out by their training that they could only perform base functions such as eating, drinking, or sleeping. There needed to be a method that could vitalize the whole body and to incorporate rational and spiritual matters as well (Britanniae, 2017).

To the ancient Greeks, a healthy mind and a healthy body were the same thing. Plato, one of the greatest Western philosophical minds, was a well-known wrestler. His name roughly translates to "broad," possibly because he was broad of both mind and body. Ancient Greek wrestling gyms known as palaestrae not only featured typical wrestling equipment such as weighted sandbags and padded mats but also classrooms where they could train their mind and spirit. This formed the start of unifying the whole body, where using physical training was a foundation to build the rest upon (Brown, n.d.).

As we can see, "mind, body, and spirit" was a way of life for the ancient Greeks, and in this book, we will further explore this unifying concept within the high intensity interval training experience (Brown, n.d.).

HIIT, the Roman Way

Let's step back in our time machine and move forward a few hundred years to the Roman Empire. Here, you will find auxiliaries, legionnaires, and generally soldiers of all types performing HIIT-style exercises, which included a great amount of hill sprinting, to keep themselves ready for war. In Machado et al.'s (2017) study, they constructed a rudimentary training regimen based on what we know of ancient Roman training techniques, carefully explaining the reasoning behind each exercise and comparing the different forms of intervals. This intense training is what separated the soldier from their competition. Roman soldiers trained to the absolute extreme, only through these kinds of extremes and or intensity is how evolution is forced and generated; further, their love of developing skills and combat strength was shown to come out of these methods.

You've probably seen the movie *Gladiator*, one of the best movies ever created, and the soundtrack brings a tear to the eye; however, I digress. A lot of movies surrounding ancient Rome take a lot of creative license with history in favor of telling a good story. Despite this, *Gladiator* is a pretty strong interpretation of what life as an ancient Roman gladiator would have been like. However, when we think of ancient Rome, we think of lavish feasts, lots of sweet wine, and hearty bread. Since gladiators made their living from fighting, they had to keep their bodies in top condition. Ancient Rome was modeled after ancient Greece in so many ways, and that includes the tetrad system we discussed earlier (Britanniae, 2017):

Day One: Preparatory workout, including strength conditioning and high-intensity workouts

Day Two: A day of high-intensity workouts, including long form exercise

Day Three: A day of rest, although lighter exercises would have been an option

Day Four: A day of moderate intensity training

If you were training at a gladiator school (ludi), you would have been subjected to a workout regimen that looked like this. Ludi customized their workout regimen, and it usually followed the above format. However, if you weren't a gladiator, you would have still been encouraged to exercise. Another concept the Romans borrowed from the Greeks was the connection between body and mind. Like Plato before him, Seneca the Younger encouraged a "return from body to mind" after exercise; he also encouraged "short and simple exercises which will tire the body with undue delay." Exercises like running, swimming, and weightlifting were options for the average, non-gladiator Roman. However, it's important to note that Seneca the Younger absolutely hated exercise, considering it a waste of time, hence the "return to the mind," which makes the case for HIIT, performing hard intense exercise for intervals of brief periods, maximizing the outcome for the shortest amount of time spent (Britanniae, 2017).

There are several other philosophers and thinkers from ancient Rome who felt differently. Marcus Aurelius, for example, subscribed to the school of Stoicism. As Stoicism became an increasingly Roman philosophy, its focus grew from mastery of the mind and emotions, to mastery of the body, mind, and soul. For a stoic like Marcus Aurelius, mastering one's physical strength was a continuous project, just as Seneca would have believed the same thing about the mind. The difference I want you to focus on, however, is that Marcus Aurelius is considered one of the greatest military minds in history.

To this day, his strategies and thoughts are taught all over the world to students of philosophy, literature, the sciences, exercise science, and many other disciplines (Britanniae, 2017).

The Romans had one of the greatest militaries in the classical world, and some of the most influential military thinkers. Their expert use of strategy was not isolated to their military. Everyone from an emperor to the common folk had some form of exercise or diet regimen that they followed to stay looking healthy. Archaeologists have built a general picture of ancient Romans and it's agreed that they were slimmer than originally thought. As we will see later on, high-intensity interval training, like what a gladiator would have done, can make drastic changes to your body. The fat burning power of HIIT keeps the metabolism burning calories and fat for days, and you build a tremendous amount of power from its exercise and practice. It's little wonder why the Romans were lithe and strong (Britanniae, 2017).

HIIT in the Modern Era and What It Can Do for You

It was only in 1785 that bodyweight exercises were integrated with standard physical education. More recently, in the 1800s, interval training was adopted by local running communities across the Western world. Of course, we have to remember that in the 1800s, they didn't have the in-depth knowledge that we have about physiology and anatomy. According to *Science of Running* (2017), interval training was developed through trial and error. This is particularly interesting, as it was often short-distance runners who took on interval training.

Nowadays, when we think of HIIT, we think of interval training which focuses on short intervals of cardio with less intensive rest periods. Most who have HIIT as part of their exercise routine will usually continue until they are too exhausted, although you will find that gyms will keep HIIT classes to 30-45 minutes, depending on the routine and intervals involved. If you want to find HIIT videos online, they will usually be around 30 minutes long. While training to exhaustion does have its place in fitness, this is not always the case for everyone; however, what this kind of training will do is allow you to test the body's limits.

Unless you are in the military or are a professional athlete, it may be that you do not access any kind of high intensity training. The same applies if you don't take it upon yourself to train at all. This lack of training can be detrimental to our health, although it can be reversed through HIIT. It may surprise you to learn that the body craves high-intensity training. You may also be surprised to learn that the need for high-intensity training is a part of our base genetic operating system ("A Misunderstanding Of High Intensity Interval Training," 2017). As the fitness industry has evolved, we have so many opportunities available to us to exercise more often. The demand for HIIT has grown over the years, and it's amazing how many people are interested in it. With such a simple format, perhaps that's what we need as the world becomes increasingly more complicated.

HIIT can be grueling, but the transformative benefits are undeniable. In a recent study, Laursen and Jenkins (2002) recorded "significant improvements in endurance performance." The study was designed to observe the effects of HIIT in endurance athletes (such as marathon runners) because endurance sports require a level of athleticism and resistance which needs to be developed through consistent practice. This study has been repeated with groups of varying abilities, and the comparisons are quite interesting. Average participants—that is to say, participants who were not professional athletes—showed remarkable improvements in their athleticism. I think it's important to note that while the original study was performed on professional athletes, it doesn't mean that the results for the average person are any less valid. Later studies concluded that HIIT can absolutely transform a person, and not just physically, but much more than ever thought; we'll get to that later.

HIIT is a full-body system which can be done with or without weighted resistance. It works by engaging your entire body leaving aftereffects for hours and days, including major boosts to hormones, fat burning properties and overall energy levels.

At the time of Laursen and Jenkins's study, there was limited information regarding HIIT. In 2002, it was seen as a fad exercise trend, but its prevalence and popularity today are proof of the opposite. As a matter of fact, more recent studies such as the one performed by Zhang et al. (2017) yielded some very interesting results. They grouped "untrained men and women" who were considered obese into one of two different types of cardiovascular exercises, one of which was HIIT; the other was MICT (moderate-intensity continuous training). Zhang et al. monitored the participants' body fat percentages across different areas where it typically congregates (trunk, abdomen, legs, buttocks, etc.) across the study period. What they found was that HIIT provided a continuous fat burning effect. While both groups lost weight and body fat, the HIIT participants had the advantage.

Zhang et al. demonstrated through this study that a 30 to 40-minute HIIT session is an effective means of fat reduction. Overall, they took both interval regimen into account, and concluded that interval training really is the way forward if you are looking to improve your metabolic rate and general health.

So, what does this mean for you? I can quote studies at you for the remainder of this book, and I will continue to refer to them as we go on, but it means nothing unless you understand what *you* personally stand to gain from high-intensity interval training.

In a word: transformation.

I understand if you think I'm bluffing. You may still think HIIT is a trendy workout only meant for people who can afford expensive gym memberships, and I don't blame you. HIIT has gathered an almost polarizing stance in the fitness community. Like with any fitness trend, there are those who swear by it and those who knock it completely. From my personal experience as a track athlete, and seeing my colleagues undertake HIIT exercises, I can promise you that I am not bluffing. I've seen the transformative effects in others and felt them in myself. My intention set for this book is to motivate you to pursue the same transformation within yourself. Later on, I am going to walk you through how to apply HIIT to three common cardio exercises: running, SPIN classes, and cycling. These exercises train the same groups of muscles in different ways which contribute to your overall performance and abilities, which will further be enhanced by high-intensity interval training.

The more HIIT you do, the more you will gain from it. Depending on how often you train, results can be seen within a month; however, internally they are felt even sooner. I mentioned that in the Zhang et al. study (2017), high-intensity interval training is the way forward to metabolic transformation. You develop within yourself an efficient fat burning machine, priming you for health beyond comprehension: a health that you will achieve.

HIIT is not just a fad exercise meant for only an elite faction of society, it is available to anyone. It has been shown time and time again to significantly transform one's cardiovascular health, insulin resistance, and overall physical well-being. As I go further in this book I will add to the physical benefits and show you it transforms your mental state and adds to your spiritual fortitude, studies will be made relevant, and we will go over various HIIT routines.

I've only just begun to scratch the surface of the physical transformation that awaits you. The second transformation you will start to feel is the mental transformation. HIIT is, as you might expect, quite grueling for the 30 minutes of exercise you do. You begin to realize how long 30 minutes is when you are performing at high intensity. And that is the first, and only, hurdle you will overcome. Once you make HIIT a regular part of your exercise plan, it becomes much more bearable, and you will soon find yourself wanting to do an extra rep or two and try to go as fast as you can. As a matter of fact, a HIIT session can quickly become your favorite part of the day.

When I talk about the mental transformation, I'm talking about the internal and external affect it has. Internally, your brain is going to start to rewire itself and become a stronger mechanism through the production of brain-derived neurotrophic factors. As a result, your mood is going to improve and you will be able to think more clearly. This is what I mean by "externally." Your thoughts become more focused and your confidence in achieving your goals skyrockets!

There are a lot of other ways in which HIIT improves your mind and brain, and I will address them throughout this book.

HIIT encourages you to practice short-term goals and helps you build confidence for your long-term ones, which will be in reach with the foundation you build for yourself through intense training. When you're doing a HIIT routine, the only person you are competing against is yourself. Just like they say in yoga, "your practice is for you." To add from Leonardo Da Vinci, "one can have no smaller or greater mastery than mastery of oneself." This leads me to the third transformation you will experience: spiritual.

To create a higher quality of life experience for yourself, we incorporate spiritual evolution—the final key in your growth—the building up of your non-physical body, and its capacity to perceive beyond the five senses including developing your athletic intuition. Intuition in general allows one to have the recognition to manage your internal processes of thought, emotions, physical, and consciousness. We will blend everything together in the execution of high-intensity interval training.

May you take from this a newfound excitement and determination to further pursue and enhance your self-development.

What we have here before us is an opportunity for grand improvement, it is only necessary to want to better yourself and the will to take the step forward. HIIT will be shown to transform one's entire being, from physical health, mental health, and spiritual health all in one unified concept. In this book, we will go over valuable studies and workout routines to give you a better idea of what awaits you in your journey with high-intensity interval training.

Chapter 1:

HIIT and Mindfulness

Stop thinking for a moment, and just focus on your breathing.

Inhale for a count of four. Focus on the sensation of the breath. Feel it expanding your rib cage and into your core. Listen to how it sounds as you inhale. Exhale for four counts. As you exhale, sigh it out as if you're letting go of everything that stresses you. Repeat five times. This is called box breathing. Box breathing is simply inhaling for a set amount of time, then holding your breath and exhaling for the same amount of time. So you would breathe for a count of four, hold for a count of four, and then exhale for a count of four, to continue with this example. Doing this will steady the breathing and calm you down. As you get used to this style of breathing, you will do it without thinking.

If you followed this simple breathing exercise, you have just practiced a basic form of meditation. This is also a common way to begin a yoga session, as it encourages the yogi to simply focus on their practice, now we want to start adding this before our exercise sessions.

Practicing meditation helps you think much more clearly and rationally about what you want to do, and how to go about it. When you practice a simple breathing exercise, you are starting to tie yourself together. What you do after, whether that's going to bed or work or getting ready for a gym session, is up to you, but a simple breathing exercise like the one I listed or a yoga practice helps you to prepare for the day ahead.

You might be wondering, "This book is about HIIT, and yoga is the complete opposite!" And you would be right because HIIT is all about getting your heart rate up and your blood pumping, and yoga is about relaxing, focusing on the breath, and letting go of everything that causes you stress. Two opposites surely can't work together, can they? Again, I understand your confusion, but allow me to explain.

We can learn a lot from how yogis prepare for their practice. HIIT and yoga actually represent two sides of the same coin: well-being. HIIT represents physical well-being, and yoga represents mental and spiritual well-being. Both encourage inner focus, both encourage strength and conditioning, and both require committed practice during the session. Just as we saw with the ancient Greeks and Romans in the introduction, training your mind and spirit is as important as training your body. For this reason, it's important to be more mindful of how we practice and to give our brains a workout as well. During this section, I am going to refer to some philosophies of mind and body which I think will help exemplify my points. At the moment, I want to continue to explore meditation.

When applied to a HIIT setting, meditation gives you a deeper awareness of your body and its needs at the time of exercising. All of us possess an innate athletic intuition to varying degrees of sensitivity. If you are not a physically active person, you might not be familiar with this term. To put it plainly, athletic intuition is a non-physical awareness of your physical body and what needs to be tuned within it, for example, amount of exercise, recovery, or where and how to heal. When you've finished your last set of a workout, it's the sense that you could push it for one more set; it also helps us determine if we're up to walking to work instead of using public transit or taking the car. Focusing on your breathing will also help you draw in more air, which translates into more oxygen for the brain. We will see in a later section the effects HIIT has on the brain.

Fitness class HIIT workouts use a combination of bodyweight and resistance training to target the whole body, section by section. Usually, they start with a light cardiovascular element which gets the heart rate going. You are also encouraged, in some cases, to use the first "block" of training to focus on the quality of the rep. Go into any gym and ask one of the trainers if it's better to do 20 high-quality reps at a slower pace, or 200 low-quality reps at a higher pace. The answer may surprise you. Performing a high-quality move, especially in the early stages of a workout, encourages a more mindful practice of the exercise and can have a better effect on the muscle group targeted. Applying this method of thinking to HIIT, you begin to understand the purpose behind the exercise. If you intend to burn fat and keep it off, you want to focus on your level of intensity; if you want to get stronger as a result of interval training, you focus on gradually increasing the resistance you apply to yourself. Your muscles will become stronger anyway, but more on that later.

When you start doing HIIT, it's going to be tempting to take the route of many low-quality reps over fewer good ones. In order to prevent injury, resist the urge. Make sure you are thoroughly warmed up and stretched before you begin. You will cause more damage to your body and experience slower progress than if you focus on quality over quantity. For an optimal workout, you should set an intention and follow through with it. If your intention is to simply burn fat and lose a few inches around your waistline, then HIIT is for you. On the other hand, if you want to condition your muscles for better strength training, you need to be mindful about the areas of your body you are training. As I keep saying, HIIT requires the practice of mindfulness. To add to that, exercise in general is a form of, and aids in, meditation. Being a full-body workout, you transition between moves very quickly, so you have to always be ready for whatever comes next.

What HIIT Can Do for the Mind

While it may have garnered a reputation for being difficult and "a new, trendy workout," you would be forgiven if you thought that HIIT was part of an exclusive or elite club of fitness enthusiasts. This is not the case. HIIT is simply a way of exercising that's available to everyone and doesn't require specialist equipment. It's 30-45 seconds of intense training, followed by 30 seconds of either rest or active recovery. The exercises are up to you, as long as they are done at high intensity. Your "recovery" period can include catching your breath, jogging on the spot, high knees, jumping jacks, or any other cardiovascular exercise which gets your blood pumping around your body.

Before I go into a more detailed explanation of the neuroscience behind high-intensity interval training, I think it's important we further look at mindfulness, its application to HIIT and what HIIT can do for your mental well-being. Something I think we all should start to understand is that, while we cannot control the events outside of our lives, we do have influence over our own minds and responses. However you choose to take control over your mind, it should be something that works for you. Whether that's seeing a professional once a week for a year or committing to a new workout routine to establish some sense of stability, that's up to you.

It's a widely accepted fact that exercise is good for the mind. Physical activity releases endorphins which make us feel happy and relieved after exercise. In a study by Jung et al. (2014), half the participants were asked to do HIIT exercises while another group were asked to do steady-state cardio. Their affective emotional responses were recorded, and Jung et al. found that the participants who did HIIT enjoyed exercising more than the participants who did steady-state cardio (Jung et al., 2014). If we can get you and more people in this mental state of enjoyment for the exercise, then more people will do it and reap major benefits. This is not the only study to come to this conclusion. In the years since this study was published, other researchers have found similar results with different sample groups, that HIIT is enjoyable thus it is continued by the individual in their self-improvement regimen.

Finding Time and Energy

Plato said, "Lack of activity destroys the good condition of every human being, while movement and methodical physical exercise save and preserve it" (Bray, 2018). We have known for a long time that exercise is great for the human body, but it's easy to forget the extent to which we need it. Depending on a variety of factors, such as your job, home life, and personal health to name a few, you might not be sure of how to best care for your body. A ballet dancer, for example, requires a level of flexibility that comes from frequent dance and yoga practice. On the other hand, an Olympic powerlifter would require a range of motion and physical control which comes from regular strength training. Boxers, due to the fast and powerful nature of the sport, need to practice HIIT exercises as a form of body conditioning; if you watch any boxing match, the jabs and strikes are often quick, powerful, and furious. This can only be achieved through high-intensity interval training. However, if you're reading this, there's a chance you aren't a ballet dancer, Olympic powerlifter, or boxer. You might be someone who wants to workout but can't find the time or motivation, or you've been given the all-clear to work out again after an injury and want to improve your athleticism. Whatever your situation, HIIT can help you.

It's difficult to find energy when you feel like you've spent it all in one place. This is why I connected yoga and meditation practice with HIIT. Plato was a wrestler as well as a teacher, and he understood the connection between mind and body. By learning to separate ourselves from our daily lives, even if it's just for a half hour three times a week, we can begin to focus on our intentions and goals. For this reason, I want you to really think about the things you want to achieve from a workout. Common goals include burning fat, toning muscle, and gaining more energy. You don't have to choose one, but keep in mind that trying to focus on too many things at once will lead to dissatisfaction, so for an optimal workout you should choose a primary focus each time you start. So, Monday could be fat burning, Wednesday muscle toning, and so on. One of my favorite things about HIIT is that it encompasses a wide range of goals and concentrates them into a single half-hour workout. That being said, there are different "flavors" of HIIT, which we will get to in just a minute.

When you work in a busy industry, are a parent, or generally struggle to find time for yourself, it feels like there aren't enough hours in the day to go to the gym and do a full workout. Spending hours in a stressful environment has been shown to be detrimental to one's mental health. You might like going to the gym, and a full workout might give you focus. It's not a bad way to spend your time. A busy day or just one bad phone call at work can leave you feeling too exhausted to go to the gym and do the same workout routine five days a week. Variety is, as they say, the spice of life. It can also be the spice of your workout.

There are multiple different "flavors" of HIIT training, one of the most popular being Tabata. This is where you recover for half the amount of time you spend exercising. So, if your exercise interval is 20 seconds, you recover for 10 seconds and repeat. Having such a small recovery window stops you from thinking about and dreading the next exercise. Instead, it pushes you to just *do* the exercise. This ultimately means you don't spend so much time at the gym. It's possible to spend an hour doing HIIT if you want to really push yourself at the gym, although this is not required. Less is more when it comes to HIIT, but as your athletic intuition increases, you will soon find yourself breaking all sorts of boundaries you never thought you had.

It may be that you find the motivation to work out in any capacity is a chore, which makes you think of working out as a chore. You get bogged down thinking about how many reps you have left, trying to conserve energy for the next exercise. Whether you're starting a new foray into fitness, or a veteran gym-goer wanting to shake up your routine, you might be struggling with motivation. High-intensity interval training has an intimidating name, and I mentioned that it can be quite grueling when you're doing it.

But, that's the magic of HIIT: the more you do it, the more motivated you become. Theoretically, you do not have to work out as much during the week as you would if you continued to go to the gym. You can get all of the fat burn and strength conditioning you need in one 20-30 minute 'super block' of high-intensity interval training. In the hours, even up to two days, following your HIIT session, your body continues to burn fat. This means that you don't have to work out nearly as often, meaning your motivation skyrockets. The motivation you gain from doing HIIT will help you follow through with attaining whatever your goals are.

You begin to see things as a challenge, and you stop comparing yourself to everyone else. Of course, you can have athletes you admire and want to emulate, but you will start to appreciate your body for what it can do for you and taking care of it through movement and methodical physical exercise is the first step toward your goals. So, I want you to really commit to yourself. When faced with challenges, we can choose to either embrace it or shy away from it. I want you to choose for yourself a half hour a day a few times a week, and just work on your goals.

Whatever goal you want to work toward, I want you to set it into motion. HIIT requires no special equipment, but you do need to have a good setup and a decent amount of space while doing it. You want to be able to get on your knees to do a donkey kick without knocking something over, and you want to lie on your back to do leg raises without hurting yourself. This is also something you need to consider if you are doing a workout video. Some workout videos are great, as they incorporate a wide variety of moves to cover the full-body range. However, some HIIT workouts have gone a step further to include a combat-based approach. This means lots of kicks and punches, so if you're going to do one of these workouts, make sure nothing's in the way. HIIT has come a long way since the early 2000s when it was simply "a hot new workout trend." Now, many athletes and gym goers recognize it for the transformative benefits it has.

Returning, then, to the art of mindfulness and its relationship to HIIT, if you practice meditation for a few minutes before you begin your HIIT session, you have the opportunity to set an intention. Setting an intention is the cornerstone of progress. It can be anything from "I will do 100 reps of exercise X in this session!" to "I will listen to my body." Once you set an intention for your workout, you will conquer the more challenging exercises and be excited for the ones that sound 'easy.'

Setting an intention doesn't have to mean thinking of your long-term goals; short-term goals are the key to a successful HIIT session, and you will quickly learn to celebrate milestones which may once have seemed like trivial markers,

Creating a Mindful Workout

There are many routes to achieving a mindful workout. You do not need to go to a yoga studio to feel a sense of calm or a gym to feel a sense of productivity. Both of these things can be achieved at home or in the area surrounding your home. A few examples of how to achieve this:

- **Create a Routine:** Plan your workouts ahead of time by choosing your "on" days and "off" days. "On" days will be days you are doing HIIT, while "off" days will be dedicated to recovery. Which days of the week those happen to be are completely up to you.

- **Start:** Whether you want to start with an advanced-level workout or you want to ease yourself in with something low impact, it doesn't matter as long as you start. The only way you are going to know if something will work or feel good is if you do it. HIIT is one of those things that feels scary at first, but once you start doing it, you start to love it.

- **Be Present:** I know how this sounds but being present doesn't just mean being physically in the room. It means knowing you are in the room, being present mentally as well as physically. Take a few moments to do the breathing exercise I went over at the start of this section, observe your surroundings, and really be mentally aware of them.

- **Set Your Intention:** Setting an intention for your workout maximizes the effects. Focus on the intensity of the block if you want to burn fat and the quality of the reps if you want to improve your strength. Always make sure that you are exercising in a way that is safe and sustainable. After a workout, you should check in with yourself to see if you've met your intention and choose an area to work toward next time.

- **Clear Your Workout Space:** A messy workout space can be a nightmare. You may not have much room to work with at home, so make sure the surrounding area is free of clutter. Your workout space can include the world outside.

Find hills or stairs to sprint up, and make sure that nothing is in your way so you avoid injury.

- **Notice How Your Body Feels:** It can be tempting to "play through the pain," but this is how injuries happen, and progress is lost. HIIT is, by definition, intense. If you feel a twinge in your shoulder, or your calves start to scream, dial back on the intensity, or change the exercise so that you are protecting yourself. If you start to feel fatigued but not injured, then try pushing through the last couple of reps and take a longer break if needed.

- **Take Stock of Your Thoughts and Emotions:** Your body isn't the only part of you that will react to your workout. Take a few deep breaths and imagine you're being scanned, noting all of the emotions that crop up for you. Do you feel excited? Could you handle another session immediately after? Are you tired and wanting a nap? This is another benefit of practicing mindfulness as part of your workout: you get to know your own mind as well as the limits of your body.

A common misconception about interval training is that the number of reps matters more than the time and effort you put into it. In fact, it's the other way around. Since interval training works in a work:rest ratio, you quickly find yourself focusing on the quality of your reps as opposed to the quantity. When you commit to a 30-minute HIIT session, just focus on those 30 minutes. After those 30 minutes are up, you can carry on with your day.

HIIT is a powerful transformative tool. In the next section, I will get into the neuroscience behind why it works so well. Right now, I want you to realize how clear-minded you are going to feel after a good HIIT session. You will start to feel your body and mind piecing themselves back together, and you will become more confident in your appearance and decision-making abilities. You will also find that breathing is much easier, and you will start to experience more even and deeper sleep.

We concern ourselves so much with the things that are going to happen in the future, and it's either in the form of a grandiose daydream or catastrophizing our worries. A school of Greek philosophy, Stoicism, discourages thinking of the future in this form. Instead, we should focus on the events of the moment, hour, and day ahead of us, not the concerns of the far future.

Don't concern yourself with what exercise you're going to do next, just focus on the exercise you are doing now. Embrace the knowledge that "day by day in every way you are getting better and better." This is a valuable affirmation called The Coue Method, by Emile Coue, a

French psychologist (Walker, 2019). I have included it into my life, and may it benefit you as well. This is the power of high-intensity interval training and what it can do for you.

Chapter 2:

Your Brain on HIIT

Now that we've covered the benefits of HIIT for the mind, we can begin to do a deep dive into the neuroscience of why HIIT is so beneficial. We already know that HIIT is a highly effective cardiorespiratory workout, but did you know that it can improve cognitive function? I will be including a lot of studies and throwing many terms at you which you might not be familiar with, please follow along as best you can, and do a little of your own research if you find yourself becoming overwhelmed. As fascinating as the neuroscience of HIIT is, it can get complicated. For this section, I'll do my best to make it simple and easy to understand.

A study by Mekari et al. (2020) investigated the link between HIIT and the brain. Their study had a group of participants perform HIIT exercises three times a week for six weeks, and the results were incredible. As per standard scientific method, the HIIT group were compared to a control group and a moderate-intensity training group. The HIIT group showed better improved cognitive function in specific tasks over the other two. In addition, HIIT has the potential to aid in the repair and reversal of age in cognitive functioning. Mekari et al.'s study was inspired by an earlier study by Van Gelder et al., who wanted to investigate the effects of high intensity exercise on dementia patients. While extraneous factors including genetics and environment should be taken into account, the Van Gelder et al. study reported that participants who took part in HIIT exercise were less likely to develop dementia over the 10-year reporting period (Mekari et al., 2020).

HIIT also increases your VO2 max. This is the maximum rate of oxygen your body is able to use during exercise. Put simply, the more HIIT you do, the more oxygen your body intakes and uses thus the brain gets more as a result. The Van Gelder et al. study noted that, "It was previously believed that there was a direct correlation between a high aerobic fitness level and increased levels of executive functioning" (Mekari et al., 2020) which is exactly what was discovered that indeed a direct correlation between the VO2 max levels and increased levels of executive functioning does occur. Van Gelder et al. are not the first to come to this conclusion. Kramer et al. were among the first to study this phenomenon (Mekari et al., 2020).

Neuroplasticity is the brain's ability to adapt to new information by restructuring its own functional and structural pathways. This results in increased learning and higher rates of productivity. Hotting and Roder's study (2013), which encompassed both human and animal trials, found that periods of physical exercise facilitates cognitive function. This is not just limited to learning, as neuroplasticity includes memory and recovery from injuries. By committing to HIIT, you have the opportunity to heal your body from any current and or future illness and injury.

Applying the Neurological Benefits of HIIT

I don't blame you if you came into this book thinking, "HIIT is just an intense form of exercise. Why do I need to know all of this?" For some people, exercise is just something to do, a way to be productive for a couple of hours a day, or just a way to get some time to themselves after work. However, there are people who want to take their training to the next level. Usually, those people are professional athletes like track athletes, who use HIIT to help them with sprint training to achieve their personal bests. People who run obstacle course races such as the Spartan Race or the Wolf Run incorporate HIIT into their training to improve their athleticism and make their race much more tolerable.

HIIT is a fast, easy way to skyrocket your performance and accelerate your personal fitness goals. Whether you want to run 52 marathons in a year, or you just want to burn some excess fat and tone up for the summer, you can achieve it through HIIT. I have said it before, and I will continue to say it: HIIT is for everyone. It can be done anywhere, and it can be done with no equipment. All you need to do is set your timer, set your intention, and just *start*.

You bought this book wanting to know more about transformation. HIIT is one of the few; or may I say, only exercise system which connects the mind, body, and spirit. We have already covered the effects on the mind, and now it's time to look at the science behind HIIT.

Retrain Your Brain

Now that we know how HIIT affects the mind, let's start to think about how we can apply this to our daily lives. In particular, I am going to start delving into the science behind HIIT, and why it works so well. In this section, I am going to talk about brain-derived neurotrophic factors, as well as cortisol and its role in the brain's functioning and development. I don't want to bore you by explaining them in one large chunk that you will soon forget, so I'm going to apply them in context.

I've already mentioned that exercise in general, especially HIIT, can increase one's capacity for learning, so we can start there. Surely there are new skills you've been meaning to acquire. Allow the learning process to be supplemented with intense exercise.

HIIT can help you not only retrain your brain but help you fast-track the learning process. It was previously believed that human adult brains stop being able to learn after age 35, but I think we have seen enough evidence to the opposite. Increased physical activity not only leads to an improved heart rate and better blood pressure, it also leads to increased oxygenation of the brain. This stimulates the production of brain-derived neurotrophic factor (BDNF), a protein found in the brain and the spinal cord. It's this protein which keeps your cells protected, aids in their maintenance processes, and most importantly, facilitates cell maturation. Your brain is, to put it simply, a mass of neurons constantly firing at each other. Without BDNF, your neurons remain unprotected and cannot perform properly (Martínez-Díaz, 2020).

The brain requires a lot of oxygen to keep its own metabolic processes in operation. Your brain is like a finely tuned battery. Neurons fire at each other at an incredible rate which allows the body to function in ways we have only just begun to understand. The brain knows when to use energy and when to conserve it. We already know that HIIT increases your VO2 max, which means that your brain will have a stronger, more reliable supply of oxygen. As a result, your body will function much better than if you weren't doing HIIT. Ultimately, you have given your brain an incredible gift: increased capacity. Another point to consider is the meditative benefits of high-intensity interval training. This is also known to help increase the brain's capacity as well.

Couple this with increased oxygen, and your brain becomes a force to be reckoned with in its own right.

As long as you keep doing HIIT, you will be able to continue to facilitate lifelong learning. Humans have a natural curiosity, stemming from our innate urge to learn about the world around us. This is why you see fitness influencers trying new exercises almost every day, and why your favorite sports apparel brand keeps researching and developing the next generation of sportswear. Of course, there are other reasons behind this second example, but the fact remains that not all exercise is created equal.

While there remains some uncertainty around the biological processes which relate to improved cognitive function, the one thing we are absolutely sure of is increased oxygenation. Going back to the previous section, where I discussed steady-state cardio, HIIT helps oxygenate your brain and body at a higher rate than steady-state cardio. If you enjoy spending hours on the treadmill and it works for you, that's fine. Adding variety to your workout will help you see results much quicker than if you were to do the same exercises over and over again. The brain loves variety; with HIIT, we have ample opportunity to give our brain the variety it so desperately craves.

You may not notice the change right away; it can take a few weeks to really kick in. It usually takes anywhere from 18 days to three months to break a habit and establish a new one. Start your HIIT habit today, and your future self will thank you.

The Role of HIIT in Healing: Cortisol and BDNF

HIIT can play a vital role in healing due to increased production of BDNF and reduced production of the steroid hormone, cortisol. Cortisol is released from the adrenal glands in small quantities. While it is often released with adrenaline, stimulating responses such as 'fight or flight,' cortisol stimulates the production of endorphins, the body's natural painkillers and mood stimulants. This is the reason you don't notice aches and pains immediately after a workout. As I established earlier, BDNF is key in keeping your neurons firing and working as much as they do. This facilitates neuroplasticity in the hippocampus, the epicenter of emotional response. Neuroplasticity in the hippocampus translates to improved emotional well-being (Martínez-Díaz, 2020).

This is an often-overlooked aspect of high-intensity interval training. It's not just your physical health that improves as a result of your commitment to HIIT. A few weeks after you start training, your mood begins to improve, and it's all down to the effect of HIIT on your brain. A lot of sports are rooted in winning or losing, and you start to judge your skill by how often you win, with high-intensity interval training you win every time you do it; further, with greater neuroplasticity in the hippocampus, your own brain starts to support you as you take on personal challenges and continue to exceed them and exceed them you will.

Some of this could be due to a better balance of hormones. As I mentioned above, when cortisol stimulates the production of endorphins, you start to feel good. The brain's system of rewarding us when we do something that feels good keeps us wanting to do more. In the case of exercise, we notice small things like how our movement changes, how much clearer our heads start to feel. This can be greatly attributed to the brain producing BDNF.

A study by Cahn et al. (2017) observed increased production of BDNF in participants after a three-month yoga and meditation retreat. While yoga is not HIIT, it is important we take note of the fact that regular exercise, low impact that it may be, led to increased production of BDNF. The participants, a mix of men and women across all ages and levels of fitness, reported high levels of anxiety and stress before going into the study. The study aimed to identify a correlation between exercise and production of BDNF. By the end of the three months, Cahn et al. report a "significant 3-fold increase' in participants compared to levels at the start of the study. Cahn et al. went on to conclude that BDNF played a significant role in the neuroplasticity of the campus, as I mentioned earlier (Cahn et al., 2017).

Simply put, HIIT can help you develop mentally as well as physically. One of the most common misconceptions about HIIT is that it's just for bodybuilders and gym bunnies who want to shed excess fat as soon as possible. We have seen in the studies I have shown you just how transformative HIIT can be.

I want you, now, to think of a goal. Make sure it's something attainable, like dropping a pant size or improving your breathing.

Have you set it?

Good, now you can start to work on it. Taking inspiration from Cahn et al., and give yourself three months to achieve that goal. Set the intention to do a HIIT regimen for as many days in the week as you feel comfortable doing and set up your workout space using the tips I provided earlier. That 30 minutes, however many times a week you've decided, is *your* time. It doesn't matter what your goal is, it's important that you make this commitment to yourself. Keep it up for three months, and you will start to see a change sooner than you expect.

Conclusion

The effects of HIIT on both the mind and brain are numerous, and they all come down to increased production of brain-derived neurotrophic factors. This simple protein, which does so much, can be seen as the root of all the mental benefits you can acquire through a regular HIIT regimen.

HIIT improves your cognitive functions, which leads to dramatically improved mental health. The studies which measured BDNF production before and after high-intensity interval training are just a sample of many. There are aspects that we did not yet go into which I will cover in the section on the spirit, that is your circadian rhythm and the many benefits tied to optimizing it.

Next, we are going to look at the effects of HIIT on the body. I've already covered some of the effects in the brain section for the sake of context, but now we are going to cover how HIIT can help you heal and help you look after yourself. You may or may not see the results you want in the first couple of weeks; however, they will come, and once you start to notice them, you will never look at exercise in the same way. You will never be the same.

Chapter 3:

Transformative Effects of

HIIT on the Human Body

And so we come to what might seem like the most obvious thing about HIIT: your physical transformation. It takes a couple of weeks for the changes to your physical appearance to show, but you will feel the internal effects within just a couple of days. The purpose of this section is to explore the transformative physical effects of HIIT. Aside from the obvious soreness after exercise, there are a lot of effects HIIT has on the human body. From burning excess fat for days after the exercise is complete to increased personal bests, you have a lot to look forward to.

A study by Di Blasio et al. (2014) characterized heart rate and hormonal responses to HIIT. The study was performed on "eight healthy trained men" whose testosterone levels were measured in addition to their heart rates. For the purposes of this section, we are going to focus on the heart rate and return to hormones later; in addition, I want to quickly explain that a normal, healthy heart rate should be between 60-100 bpm (beats per minute). This, of course, varies depending on how active you are, your weight, your height, and your age. A lot of factors influence it, so don't panic if you go to your doctor after a couple of weeks of doing HIIT and find that your heart rate has suddenly increased from 72 to 89. This is still considered normal and healthy (Di Blasio et al., 2014).

Di Blasio et al. gave the participants a variety of HIIT exercises, and they discovered that their heart rates increased to around the same level regardless of the type of HIIT exercise (whether it was organized or random). Getting your heart rate up during exercise is great for circulation, but it's even better for the heart, brain and lungs (Di Blasio et al., 2014).

HIIT and Lung Power

Earlier, we looked at something called "VO2 max." I'd like to revisit it and go into a more detailed exploration of how HIIT can help you achieve your physical goals. As I mentioned earlier, your VO2 max is essentially your maximum oxygen uptake, and many studies have been published with evidence supporting HIIT and its efficacy regarding cardiovascular health. Astorino et al. (2012) studied the effects in healthy young adults and noticed that all participants experienced significant physical changes.

This study is interesting. Although we know that exercise can affect your blood pressure, Astorino *et al* performed the study on healthy men and women who were already active. For this reason, it appears that blood pressure and resting heart rate were unchanged. However, the thing I would really like you to focus on is the change in VO2 max: "Data reveal that short-term HIIT improves Vo2 max, power output, and O2 pulse in active men and women" (Astorino et al., 2012).

Astorino et al. stated that while they weren't measuring *why* this sudden increase in VO2 max occurred, they put it down to *increased cardiovascular activity and more oxygen* flowing around the body. Think back to the previous section where I explained the relationship between increased oxygenation and its benefits for the brain. When we breathe, our lungs take in as much as 1.5 gallons of air. If you do high-intensity interval training on a regular basis, you can increase this to so much more and give your brain the oxygen it needs to release BDNF (Astorino et al., 2012)..

This study had a variety of methods to test the researchers' objectives. If VO2 max can be greatly enhanced by short-term HIIT, imagine what you could achieve with a long-term commitment.

While there have been a multitude of studies regarding HIIT and its relationship to VO2 max and power output, there have been as many studies examining HIIT and lung health. We have some evidence that it can help improve the well-being of recovering lung cancer patients, and we also have evidence that lung health improves in general as a result of high intensity interval training. A study by Enright et al. (2006) examined the effect of high-intensity training on the muscular strength of the lung.

Maximum Inspiratory Pressure (MIP) was measured in relation to a short-term course of high-intensity training. When compared to the baseline at the start of the study, participants showed a 41% increase in MIP at the end of the study. Enright et al.'s study concluded that high-intensity training significantly improves the overall health and strength of lungs, reporting that participants' lungs were much stronger after consistent high-intensity training than they were before (Enright et al., 2006.

For people who struggle with their breathing, such as asthmatics and allergy sufferers, HIIT could be a highly effective tool. If you are an endurance athlete, training for your next marathon or obstacle course race, you could significantly improve your chances and stamina by doing high intensity interval training a couple of times a week.

HIIT and Your Nervous System

Let's return, for a moment, to Laursen and Jenkins. Back in 2002, they compiled a paper which took all of the research at the time and created a scientific case for HIIT. If you made it this far in the book, you will have seen how much I love quoting studies. In Laursen and Jenkins's paper, they listed all sorts of sources which, at the time, spearheaded the popularity of HIIT. Back in 2002, when people heard the words "backed by science," they flocked toward it. Most workout trends and fads die out after a couple of years, but it's the ongoing scientific fascination with high-intensity interval training that has ensured its longevity, which has endured from ancient times, and for this reason it will continue.

The age-old adage that "exercise keeps you healthy" has a long history of scientific evidence. Back in 2017, Nair et al. studied the effects of high-intensity interval training on equal groups of young and older volunteers. The goal of the study was to see how exercise affects the body on a molecular level. By testing the levels of protein produced after exercise, Nair's team discovered that the group who performed HIIT exercises had more active mitochondria. If you've ever sat in a biology class and studied cell anatomy, you will have heard that the mitochondria are the powerhouse of the cell. Nair et al. also tested participants through cycling and strength training and determined that each exercise has its benefits (Cell Press, 2017).

Mitochondrial strength is the basis of a healthy nervous system. Without mitochondrial biogenesis, most of the bodily functions we experience on a daily basis would not be possible. If we cast our minds back to VO2 max and its effects on endurance performance, we start to build a picture of how the mitochondria can help us transform and achieve our optimal performance.

Adenosine triphosphate (ATP) is a nucleic acid used as the energy source for mitochondrial biogenesis. Our cells use it as a form of currency for synaptic signaling, muscular contraction, and active transport. This is just a sample of what little nucleic acid can do.

High-intensity interval training, as we have seen, improves your mitochondrial strength and gives you a better idea of what your body is capable of. As a result, your athletic intuition increases. This is how you know when to give your body an extra push, as well as when to hold back in training. For the moment, I want you to reflect on your personal goals. When you are working out, it could be to improve your mental health, your physical health, or just to get a couple of hours to yourself. A wide variety of transformations can occur as a result of HIIT.

As we age, our mitochondrial capacity steadily decreases. This means that our cells stop producing the proteins and energy sources we need. Nair et al. found that high-intensity interval training effectively rejuvenated participants' ribosomes. These are the 'building blocks' of cellular proteins. It has been shown time and time again that exercise is good for us in so many ways, but we rarely stop to think beyond "I will go for a run three times a week" or "strength training will reshape my body." While running is a great cardiovascular exercise, and strength training is good for muscle growth, we end up exercising ineffectively and cause our bodies more harm later in the future. For this reason, we have to be more attentive to how we choose to help our bodies.

You often hear bodybuilders and weightlifters talk about "arm day" and "leg day" or even "shoulder day." While it's tempting to work every single part of your body every single day you go to the gym, you have to remember that your body requires rest to process everything that you are putting it through. This is something I am going to keep saying because it's far too easy to get hurt by overworking ourselves. One of the great things about HIIT is that it *does* work the whole body, but you exercise in efficient chunks so that no single part of your body is overworked (Cell Press, 2017).

Adding high intensity interval training to your regimen three times a week can significantly accelerate your performance. On a molecular level, your body will produce much more energy, power your nervous system and improve your athleticism. Everything will just fall into place and build on itself, the nervous system will adapt to the intense stress and become that much stronger, which will even further lead to your cardiovascular, brain, and immune health.

HIIT and Your Hormones

Human growth hormone (HGH or GH) is secreted by the pituitary gland. It is responsible for increasing muscle mass and decreasing body fat. During puberty, we secrete more of it to stimulate linear growth (height) in children. You might already be able to tell that HGH is an important hormone. Studies into the concentration and effects of HGH after HIIT exercise are still ongoing, but we can gain some useful insights from the few studies we do have. For example a study performed by Loughborough University, U.K. found that "Metabolic responses were greater after the 30 seconds [of sprinting] than after the 6 second sprint. The highest measured mean serum HGH concentrations after the 30 s sprint were more than 450% greater than after the 6 s sprint" (Stokes et al., 2004). This occurred when sprinting at near full capacity for 30 seconds. We can therefore infer that HIIT ideally should be performed above 80% capacity, as this is when we see HGH levels rise 500% or higher. Here, we can see that sprinting is very ideal. I personally use it, however HIIT in general is a powerful stimulus for hormone secretion and regulation.

As an adult, human growth hormone helps stimulate muscle growth. It won't make us taller, but it can help make our bones thicker and help us develop strength. That being said, increased muscle mass does not equate to more strength. This is what strength training is. Abderrahman et al. (2018) found some evidence that HGH production increased toward the end of a long-term HIIT regimen. It's important to note that the Abderrahman et al. study lasted for seven weeks and was performed on 24 male participants. As we continue with HIIT long term, the beneficial effects start compounding. When you hear about the importance of a rest day when going to the gym, it's not only to allow your body the chance to rest and process the workout, it's to help your recovery hormones do their jobs. You will only see an increase in muscle mass if HGH is allowed the space to work properly, where it contributes significantly to anti-aging and total healing (Abderrahman et al., 2018).

A lot of studies done in regard to the stimulation of human growth hormone revolve around men and adolescent males, with limited information on how it affects women after a bout of HIIT. Of the evidence we do have, it seems that the fat-burning potential of HIIT is higher in women, likely due to a higher average body fat percentage. The one study I could find which has any measure of integrity in this area is the Copeland et al. study (2002), which studied a broad range of women between ages 19 and 69. You could consider this a bit of a landmark study because it so thoroughly tested female hormones from such a wide age range. What Copeland et al. found was that secretion of human growth hormone, as a result of a six-week course of high-intensity interval training, was much higher than any of the studies I could find which focused on males. Where Abderrahman et al. showed that HGH increased gradually in men, Copeland et al. found that HGH levels had a higher increase in response to endurance exercises than to any of the other exercises in the study group (Copeland et al., 2002).

Applying this understanding of HIIT to our everyday lives, I would like you to understand that HIIT will not help you grow taller. Instead, I want you to focus on the potential HIIT has to help you become stronger and more confident in your body. When you perform HIIT exercises, not only will your body start to work at its peak performance, this energy will continue into your recovery period. Rest and recovery days are so important after exercise for all the reasons I stated earlier. If you want to do some active recovery to help your muscles loosen up, go with a light jog or some yoga. This will help with any aches and pains you may be feeling without causing damage to the body. Moving on from this, you will most likely notice the changes to your body in the rest periods. After a HIIT workout, once you've recovered and caught your breath, you are going to start feeling warm. Rest assured that this is completely normal, it's just your body responding to the exercise and working to help itself heal and feel good. This is just the beginning of your transformation.

HIIT and the Metabolism

Your base metabolic rate is the rate at which you burn calories when resting. An average adult human male burns between 2,000-2,500 calories a day, and an average adult human female burns between 1,800-2,000 calories a day. A lot of factors go into determining your base metabolic rate, including, but not limited to age, physical activity level, body fat percentage, muscle mass, gender, hormones, and genetics. You may hear about the latest craze in the diet and wellness industry being pills and teas which "boost thermogenesis." Thermogenesis is simply a by-product of calories burning and it does not need to be boosted with tea or pills. So, whenever you see the words "boosts thermogenesis" at a health food store, just ignore it. This perfectly normal and functional process is being used to dupe you into the latest unsustainable health craze.

With this in mind, I would like you to know one important thing about thermogenesis: it also increases as a result of exercise. This is what helps you continue to burn fat after a workout at the gym. Strength training helps shape your body by toning targeted muscle groups, HIIT shapes your body by keeping the muscle gains and allowing it to continue to burn calories and, therefore, fat for up to two days after a workout. Put simply, the more heat you create through exercise, the more fat you burn. You sweat because your body is trying to cool itself down, but you feel warm because your body is burning so many extra calories.

Because high-intensity interval training is so, well, *intense*, you end up burning more calories through thermogenesis. As a matter of fact, you could burn up to nine times more fat with HIIT than with any other workout. Astorino et al. (2018) led a study to evaluate this. This study was an exploration into the results of a four-week course of HIIT compared to sprint interval training (SIT), and it has paved the way for more studies in the years since it was published. This study showed no significant increase in base metabolic rate after HIIT, but there was an incredible increase in base metabolic rate following bouts of SIT. After sprint interval training, the participants' base metabolic rates increased by up to twice the magnitude of HIIT. Another thing Astorino et al. noticed was the increase in oxygen uptake in addition to small changes in body fat percentage. All of this after just four weeks of sprint interval training. While this is an area which is still under scientific investigation, these results are absolutely incredible. One last thing I want you to take from this study is that SIT was considered "a time-efficient stimulus" to base metabolic rate after the four-week study, which means that the participants got more out of it for the time they put in. I want you to remember this because, later on, I am going to start walking you through sprint training (Astorino et al., 2018).

One study to come out as a result of the Astorino et al. study was the Petrofsky et al. study (2011), which examined the effects of 10-minute rounds of HIIT. While not the half hour I'm suggesting, if you enjoy going to the gym, adding an extra 10 minutes of HIIT to the end of your workout could help amplify everything you have done. Something important to note is that the Petrofsky et al. study was very well controlled, everything from the diet to water consumption was monitored during this study. The participants, a mix of men and women, showed an increase in base metabolic rate, burning an average of 62 extra calories an hour for four hours after performing a six-minute HIIT regimen. As I mentioned, the study was highly controlled to avoid weight gain and loss as this study was purely to measure the effects of a short HIIT bout on the base metabolic rate. Even with this in mind, the base metabolic rate continues to increase and burn at a steady rate (Petrofsky et al., 2011).

For the purposes of this book, and to help you understand the powerful transformative effects this will have, I want you to think about how this could affect you and your fitness goals. If you only do HIIT three times a week, you could achieve your goals more effectively than if you were to go to the gym and workout five days a week. We live in a busy world, and if you work in a job that demands a lot of hours, it can be hard to imagine how you could fit a full workout into your schedule. While a half hour three times a week might not seem like much in the way of a workout, and I understand if you're not convinced, it's better than doing nothing. One thing I am going to keep repeating is that HIIT can be done anywhere. If you have stairs close to home, you can do stair sprints; if there's a park or a running track near where you live, you can do sprint intervals; at home, you can clear a space and do a HIIT workout video three times a week. Through intense interval exercise, you can efficiently burn fat with increased metabolism and help build and maintain muscle in short periods of time.

How HIIT Will Transform Your Body

Another interesting study I want to direct your attention to is the Kong et al. (2016) study on the effects of HIIT on obesity. The researchers wanted to focus on body composition, blood glucose and "relevant systemic hormones." Like I said earlier, it will take a couple of weeks before you start to see your body shape change. That being said, you *will* feel your body start to change on the inside. Kong et al. discovered that their participants' body composition changed significantly in the 5-week period they were asked to perform HIIT exercises. The same study also reported that fasting glucose—your blood sugar after an overnight fast (for example, when you wake up after sleeping for eight hours)—was significantly lower than the control study. Insulin is the hormone which maintains your blood sugar level. Regular exercise is known to help with your blood glucose, and thanks to the Kong et al. study, we can see that HIIT is an incredibly effective method of maintaining your blood sugar (Kong et al., 2016).

We are now going to briefly revisit the effects of HIIT on cortisol. Chronically high levels of cortisol can have detrimental effects on your health. It's known as the stress hormone for a reason. Zoreta-Ortega et al. (2019) studied a small group of male college athletes with the intention of analyzing their blood plasma levels. In doing this, they would determine the concentration of cortisol and testosterone. Zoreta-Ortega et al. noted that there is some controversy surrounding the effects of HIIT on a person's hormone levels. While the sample size was small, this study inspired a lot more research into this very area. For the purposes of this section, I want us to briefly consider the implications of this study (Zoreta-Ortega et al., 2019).

While Zoreta-Ortega et al. observed no change to the concentration of testosterone immediately after exercise, they noticed that 12 hours after exercising, testosterone levels had increased and appeared to be more stable than when samples were first taken. They also observed that cortisol levels remained consistent throughout each sample. But this is just how HIIT affects the hormone levels in men. Copeland et al. (2002) observed that, following a protocol of HIIT, women between the ages of 19-69 experienced an increase in all hormones being tested for, including testosterone, serum growth hormone, plasma lactate, and estradiol (an estrogen steroid hormone which is active in the female reproductive system). There are significant differences between these two studies. For example, Zoreta-Ortega et al. used a small sample size entirely consisting of men in the same age group, while Copeland et al. studied a larger group of women across different age groups.

To add some more information on testosterone we know that high speed sprinting even for short bouts of six seconds increases testosterone production (Stokes et al., 2004).

With this in mind, we begin to get a larger picture of how high-intensity interval training can be beneficial across the spectrum. Hormone levels fluctuate during exercise, but in the hours following a period of HIIT, our hormone levels start to achieve a sense of balance.

Our bodies start to cool down and become stronger in the process. High-intensity interval training not only makes us healthier, but it makes us more balanced.

Conclusion

I think it's safe to conclude that high-intensity interval training is transformative not just for the mind and brain but for the body as a whole. While HIIT will not help us shed the pounds immediately, it will change our composition so that we burn more fat for longer periods of time, in addition to priming our muscles and brains for better functionality with the help of beneficial hormone release. In addition, HIIT helps keep our hormones balanced, while improving our personal output which is measured by VO2 max. This is the athletic potential we are assisted in achieving, transforming us physically in ways we wouldn't expect.

Chapter 4:

HIIT and Recovery

So, you've finished your workout, and you're feeling great. Maybe you're at the gym and want to get in some extra strength training. Or, you're at home and just want to unwind with some herbal tea and a couple of episodes of your favorite TV show. Congratulations! You did it! You completed a session of high-intensity interval training and now you get to enjoy the benefits. This is the easy part, just letting your body rest, and knowing that the last half hour is going to help change you for the better.

What can you look forward to now that you're resting? I've spent the last few chapters going over the scientific basis of high-intensity interval training, and its effects on the body. For the purposes of this chapter, we're going to take it light, and give you a rundown of all the things you can expect in the coming days and weeks, in terms of changes to your body and mind. Along those lines, we are also going to start touching on the spiritual nature of high-intensity interval training. This is something which people often ignore when they think of exercise. Not just with HIIT, but with everything including yoga and a simple jog.

We know that exercise is good for us, and as with all good things, it's true that you can have too much of it. Too much running can lead to damaged joints, too much strength training—or even just using weight you aren't yet ready for—can potentially cause irreparable muscle damage. Ballet dancers often suffer from plantar fasciitis or sesamoiditis; the former is a painful inflammation of the heel; the latter is chronic inflammation of the bones beneath the big toe. Health problems can arise from overexercise, so it's important that we learn when to pull back. Recreational exercise is best enjoyed in moderation, so we have to learn a little thing called athletic intuition.

Athletic intuition requires you getting to know your body intimately, not on a physical or external level, but to start feeling what is happening to your body on the inside. Earlier, I mentioned a trick actors use when they're preparing for a role, the imaginary body scan. Imagine you are in a body scanning machine—maybe it's an MRI scanner or you could be lying on top of the copier at your workplace—and start to mentally scan your body, being aware of all the aches and pains your body throws at you. Does your shoulder twinge when you move it a certain way? Do your knees ache when you bend them too far? Does your groin hurt when you're sitting into a jump squat?

Doing a mental scan like this gives us an idea of our body's limitations and ways to circumvent them, preventing injuries and further pain along the line. Injuries as a result of too much exercise take longer to heal than an injury sustained from conscious, moderate exercise. One of the best things about high-intensity interval training is you start to develop an innate sense of awareness in your body. Keeping in line with this, I would like you to remember what I said about brain-derived neurotrophic factors and their effects on the brain. A part of this innate awareness comes from better optimized cognitive functioning. While we want to train as hard as we possibly can, we start to understand what we're comfortable doing.

Take a standard "block one" HIIT routine, performed twice over at a 45:15s work:rest ratio:

- Jumping jacks

- Rest

- Burpees

- Rest

- Mountain climbers

- Rest

- Jump squats

- Rest

- Plank jacks

As you may have noticed, I have given a series of exercises which require a lot of energy in a very short space of time. The first time you try a HIIT routine like this, you will feel absolutely exhausted, maybe wanting a bit more, but you will be in dire need of a relaxing tea break or maybe a long shower to help ease your muscles. Now, think about doing the same routine the next day, and certain areas of your body might start to throb with pain.

When exercising, no matter if it's HIIT, cycling, running, or any kind of sport, you have to make sure your body is up to the task. That's why rest days are so important. Whether you prefer to do two days in the gym and one rest day or five days in a row and have the weekend as your recovery time. Resting gives our bodies an opportunity to process what it just went through and allows us the opportunity to listen to, and understand, what it needs.

High-intensity interval training, as the name describes, requires your maximum effort from start to finish. You put a lot of effort in for what seems like minimal results, but I promise you that this is not the case. After a few weeks of continuous high-intensity interval training, you will start to notice how your body, mind, and spirit are changing for the better. I won't spend too long on the studies this time, I promise. Instead, I want to excite you about the things you have to look forward to.

First of all, let's look at how your body is going to change after your training and maximizing your recovery. I have already gone through the studies and explained how hormones affect us and how the cells react to exercise. We can now start to apply this knowledge to our daily lives, and you can start to envision the future of your health and well-being.

Continuous and consistent high-intensity interval training strengthens the central nervous system, largely through mitochondrial density. It's through mitochondrial biogenesis that our cells develop energy and power. When you perform HIIT exercises as a consistent rate, allowing adequate time for your body to relax and recover, you will begin to notice that you have much more energy than you previously had. This is all down to these tiny little powerhouses in our cells, moving faster and developing more ATP to facilitate all of our bodily processes. As the weeks go by, you will be able to train harder and faster, developing a capacity for HIIT that you had never previously imagined including developing a more productive recovery rate.

The next physical change you have to look forward to will take a little bit longer than you might expect. People take up high-intensity interval training because they think it will shed the pounds a lot faster than slower, moderate intensity training. While you can lose a lot of weight with HIIT, the process happens internally before you start to see any exterior results. On the inside, your metabolism will burn fat at a much faster rate than normal, which will ultimately change your body composition. It's entirely possible for you to be the same weight and just have a different body fat percentage a month after you start doing HIIT. If this happens to you, *keep going*. It's only a matter of time before your waist starts to tighten up and your pants start to fit a little looser.

Finally, let's look at all the incredible things you have to look forward to mentally. Exercise has been shown many times to improve our cognitive functions. Depending on the type of exercise you do, you stand to improve a wide variety of physical skills. Because you're given so little time to think about how to do the exercises, high-intensity interval training can help you improve your coordination. Through consistent training, you will begin to notice that your mind is much clearer than before. A large part of this is due to increased oxygenation of the brain, which will stimulate the production of brain-derived neurotrophic factors as well as the powerful recovery and healing that happens once HIIT becomes a staple in your life. This healing affects your total being. An interesting side effect of mental healing is that you will start thinking about things in a deeper way, taking the time to understand and appreciate, thus developing your decision-making and further compounding the transformation within you.

Remember, high-intensity interval training can be very hard on the body. I cannot stress enough the importance of proper recovery and rest. If you feel you need an extra day, do not hesitate to take it—it will mean you can do a better workout later. Recovery will include any time off and relaxation, as well as incorporating active recovery which includes, for example, light stationary cycling, slow jogging, or light swimming to help heal muscles and flush out toxins.

Incorporating Sauna and Steam Rooms

I know what you're thinking. "First yoga, now saunas & steam rooms? Are you sure this is a book about HIIT?" HIIT is exercise, just like running on the treadmill and lifting weights. As I've been saying, after exercise, you need to recover. One of my favorite methods of recovery is to use the sauna or steam room at my local gym. If you have a steam or rain shower, you have an idea of the level of relaxation and unwinding a sauna or steam room can provide. There's just something about sitting in a foggy room, inhaling steam and letting your mind do whatever it wants. We already know about the benefits of steam breathing when we're sick: it dislodges mucus and clears our airways, allowing clearer breath. I don't think I need to tell you that this is amazing for the brain too, since more air in the lungs means more oxygen for the brain! Further studies also show that sauna usage increases HGH, which only adds to the benefits the HIIT workout did for you in the first place (The Rugby Republic, 2016).

A good session in the sauna or steam room is also a great communal place. I'm not much of a talker in there unless I know the people I'm with well, but it's lovely seeing people talk and decompress together. This sort of thing is also pretty great for the mind.

Speaking of the mind, saunas and steam rooms release some pretty amazing endorphins which aid in stress relief and help us relax. The heat from saunas or steam rooms benefit us in more ways than just helping dislodge mucus from our airways. The heat can cause blood vessels to dilate which increases blood flow as a result of our body temperatures rising. With this increase in blood flow, endorphins and hormones such as testosterone and HGH get around our body much faster, which streamlines and speeds up the healing process.

Once you're done with your workout, I would recommend setting yourself up in the sauna or steam room for a good total time of about a half hour (it does not need to be done in one sitting) to really absorb all the benefits it has to offer, such as muscle relaxation and the elimination of lactic acid. A good sauna or steam can really flush your body of all the things that can cause it harm. The best time to enjoy this is around midday or early afternoon because endorphins flowing about your body can be great, they don't always promote a good night's sleep. Using a sauna or steam room a little earlier in the day will allow your endorphins to gradually taper down moving into the evening; when bedtime rolls around you'll find yourself sleeping as deeply as a bear in winter.

Sauna or steam bathing is a very good way to improve your overall health through utilizing heat and sweating, which is the body's way of cooling us down when we're too hot, sweat being 99% water, and you can use it as a measure of how hydrated you are. So, the more you sweat, the better hydrated you are. This is why I will always recommend saunas and steam rooms to anyone and everyone. A good sauna or steam room session will help you sweat out all sorts of muck from your skin, including skin cells, leading to a vibrant and healthy skin complexion even after only a few sessions.

Of course, there are risks to using a sauna or steam room. Most issues—such as dizziness, lightheadedness, extreme thirst, and headaches—are usually the result of dehydration. To prevent this, make sure you go into a sauna/steam room well-hydrated and don't stay inside for too long. Additionally, like I recommended at the start of the book, you should consult a medical professional before using a sauna or steam room. This goes double if you suffer from a chronic illness such as diabetes or kidney disease, since you might be more at risk of becoming dehydrated. As many benefits as there are to using a sauna and or steam room after a workout, your medical health must come first.

Conclusion

Making a significant commitment to yourself often feels scary. It's easy to commit to a new project at work or to dinner plans with your best friend because those things are in the service of others. When you choose to make a commitment to yourself, it requires an admission of deserving to let go and embrace changes that you need in your life. High-intensity interval training helps us do this. Transitions between exercises are often quick and rest periods are short, so we stop overthinking and just start *doing*. We become much more mindful as a result of looking inward and addressing the things we need to change. Getting fit and healthy is a worthy goal, something we can all accomplish, and can be accomplished in just a half hour a few times a week.

Saunas and steam rooms are also an amazing way to relax after a good workout session. They promote the release of endorphins and beneficial hormones which help you feel good as well as doing wonders for your circulation. This helps with your stress levels in addition to improving your body's healing capabilities. Your health will also improve as a result of sauna usage, in particular the health of your skin. Through deep sweating, your skin becomes cleaner and healthier; add to this the increased blood flow enhancing your skin's life cycle, helping your skin to become stronger and feeling younger. Finally, I cannot stress enough the importance of remaining hydrated before and after going in.

You deserve to take this chance on yourself and feel like a whole new person. To become a new person, these opportunities don't present themselves often. Take it while it's fresh in your perception and start. A solid part of your recovery should always include embracing how much you have achieved in such a short space of time.

When you finish your last rep, you might hate yourself, and your body might hate you for putting it through so much, but when you wake up the next morning and perform recovery stretching, you will feel like a brand-new person. Soon, your results will start to appear so fast that by the time you get many months into your training, you will experience a phenomenal improvement in your overall health and fitness.

Chapter 5:

HIIT and Spiritual

Transformation

In order to prepare us for the next couple of chapters, let's start to think a bit more about the spiritual level of high-intensity interval training. Spirituality is more than a person's relationship with their god or gods. A spiritual person looks within for guidance. They're a mindful person who is in tune with their body, mind, and the world around them. It's the development of your non-physical self. They take the time to appreciate what life has to offer and the people around them. When I talk about spirituality as a result of exercise, I am talking about the connection between mind and body which transcends the physical and mental benefits of high-intensity interval training. Exercise, in so many ways, is a form of meditation. Very intense exercise can help aid and increase capacity for meditation, which is an invaluable tool I would recommend adding into your life.

Think about the goal you set a couple chapters ago. As you work toward it through HIIT, you will start to notice some incredibly specific changes which you were not expecting. For example, yoga has been shown time and again to improve the quality of sleep and relax the body. HIIT works in the same way. As you lie down to sleep, you will likely fall asleep much faster, and have a deeper quality of sleep which increases dream state or REM (rapid eye movement). Entering the dream state is a way for the brain to process the events of the day. Even if you don't actively dream, your brain is still working away in the background, like the antivirus on your laptop, processing everything that has happened so you can wake up feeling rejuvenated and refreshed. If you do dream, it further allows you to process your life and the way you fit into it. Regardless, if that isn't for you, deep sleep is very beneficial which will allow your body to heal much faster. After intense exercise, our body responds exceptionally well to sleep, further enhancing your healing and transformation.

With transformation, we start thinking about our perceptions of the boundaries that have been created for us and or we created ourselves, we realize breaking them is possible. What meditation offers us is that power and gives us the ability to look inward and let go of the things that are bothering or do not serve us, intense progression and a beautiful state of mindfulness follows. The ability to meditate deeply as a result of high-intensity interval training will further expand your limits. You will bear witness to your training reaching maximum efficiency almost every session. You will break through plateaus and your boundaries, and you will break your personal records and set ever increasing personal goals. One of the reasons track athletes perform at maximum capacity is because they constantly find themselves breaking their old boundaries and setting new limits. This is a further example of the power of incorporating sprinting into your own regimen. Another incredible thing you will discover as you continue to train is you will realize you have no limits but the ones you set for yourself. This will be further amplified by your athletic intuition which will dramatically increase along with your progress, contributing to a form of confidence beyond your imagination.

After examining the spiritual nature of high-intensity interval training, I would like you to do a quick mental scan right now. Assess how you are feeling, recognize any thoughts and concerns that crop up, and just let them disappear. Listen to your body and get an idea of how you are feeling internally. If you're reading this book, unsure about whether high-intensity interval training is right for you and wanting to know what you stand to gain, I want you to think about the person you want to be in the months to come. Do you want to feel less stressed? Would you like to feel more confident with your appearance? Are you ready to make a significant change to your lifestyle? Are you ready to achieve greatness within yourself?

If the answer to any of these questions is "yes," then you should absolutely try HIIT. You may feel like you have tried everything under the sun to eliminate brain fog, improve your general health and well-being, and bring yourself into balance, but until you have tried HIIT coupled with meditation, you haven't tried everything. There is a whole host of scientific evidence to back up the various points I have made throughout the last few chapters, and there is more to come.

Once you make the commitment to high-intensity interval training, the journey over the months is the beautiful part, not the end goal, it is how you get there, and what you learn along the way that matters. These memories and experiences you develop will continue to be remembered and acted further upon in your life—this is your process of transformation.

As I mentioned before, one of the things we tend to forget about exercise is how it transforms us spiritually, how it advances our emotional well-being, and how a state of inner peace overtakes you, all from intense exercise. The reason many yoga-types are so "at peace" and relaxed is because they practice the art of meditation when doing yoga, which helps them become more present and focused on the now rather than the future.

In a study exploring the perceptual and cardiovascular responses to high-intensity interval exercises, Malik et al. (2019) made some intriguing discoveries. While the study was primarily focused on adolescents, I think adults can learn quite a lot about gaining enjoyment from exercise. Their research indicates that the higher the level of intensity, the more enjoyment felt in the recovery period. Malik et al. (2019) also appear to have noticed that enjoyment was felt *during* exercise, not just after (Malik et al., 2019).

One explanation for this is that our motivation builds as a result of exercise and the powerful hormones that are released. High-intensity interval training starts off as difficult, but as you continue to do it, you start to turn it into a challenge. If you were to do a yoga class, you would hear the teacher say some variation of the words, "Do not follow others' practice, use this time to explore your own body and focus on your own practice." The same principle is true of a group HIIT class at the gym. You might take a look over your shoulder to see what position everyone else is in to make sure you're on the right track; however, ultimately it is only a competition against yourself, you start winning over yourself, and this success envelopes you in much to feel good about.

As Malik et al. found with their study, one's perception changes with the intensity and length at which they do high intensity interval exercise. The participants of this study started to see HIIT as more of a personal challenge rather than a game to win, like they would with a team-based sport where winning and losing are expected outcomes. With HIIT you realize you never lose. While a little friendly competition is fine now and again, you are ultimately in control of your own choices and actions. On some level, you may feel stuck. These sorts of mental blocks can be cleared. It's when we start to push ourselves—mentally, physically, and spiritually—that we begin to break out of the prisons we built for ourselves (Malik et al., 2019).

We tell ourselves stories of the people we are, and we take on someone else's perceptions. If the people in your life see you as easy going, a pushover, or set in your ways, you might start to think of yourself as such. It's difficult to admit, but we absorb a lot of information about ourselves through how others perceive us. Whether this is in what they tell us directly, their behavior toward us, or the responsibilities we are entrusted with at work or home, we build a picture of ourselves, little by little.

This begins to shape our actions. You might take fewer risks, like not going for that promotion at work or signing up for that race. This all stems from the fear of how people will perceive us after. If you fail at getting that promotion, you might worry that your co-workers will think less of you and make fun of you behind your back. By signing up for that race, the people who love you might inundate you with the risks associated with training and running the race from the second you press the sign-up button.

When you start doing high-intensity interval training, this all becomes irrelevant. The mental prisons of others shatter, in as much that it will not affect the way you conduct yourself or the way you view yourself, you stand solid. Starting something new, like a workout regimen or a goal you want to achieve, is a stepping-stone to a new you. Use high-intensity interval training, allow it to assist you in pushing your own boundaries, pushing the envelope of what's possible and do not allow others perceptions of their limits to be placed on you; further, do not place limits on yourself, obtain the necessary strength you need from your spiritual transformation that you gain from intense training, to carry you through life.

Thinking about all the ways you can and should apply these principles to your daily life. If you feel limited at your job, it might be because you have boxed yourself in as "the person always on the lowest rung of the ladder." At home, if you feel like all the domestic responsibilities have fallen to you, it might be because that's what you think is expected of you. It might be that you never pursued what you truly wanted to do in life. I want you to know that none of these scenarios and many more are the case; you have the power to break out of it. All you need to do is commit to making one change. Add high-intensity interval training into your life! By pushing yourself physically to your maximum, you will reap the amazing benefits the physical has to offer; in addition, it also translates into phenomenal mental benefits and spiritual changes. All of these combined promote and ensure lifelong transformation, transformation you deserve and will attain!

How the Spartans Trained

You might be familiar with the movie *300*, about the 300 Spartans who faced the Persians at the Gates of Thermopylae. While the movie takes a significant amount of creative license with regard to historical events, I think it's important that we look at the Spartans to see how our environment affects our understanding of health and wellness. I want these next sections to be about unifying the mind and body with the spirit. For this purpose, I want to continue to look at the unification of it all.

To examine the relationship between spirit and body, we will look to the Spartans. Back in 480 BC, around the time of the battle of Thermopylae, Sparta was a Greek city-state. Ancient Greece had a fierce enough training regimen for the body and mind, but ancient Sparta was something else altogether. When you think of a Spartan warrior, you likely picture a super buff man with washboard abs and bulging biceps weathering leather underpants, a blood-red cape, and not much else apart from, perhaps, a pair of sandals.

As far as we know, this is not an inaccurate picture of what a Spartan warrior would have looked like. A young boy would have started training in a Spartan agoge (or program) at as young as seven years old. The details of Spartan training would shock you because we would consider it extremely traumatic. However, Sparta was a military state, and they trained their warriors young and with brutality to prepare them for the brutality of life in the Spartan military. In brief, a Spartan boy's parents would turn him over to the state, and he would be assigned to a company at the agoge where he would live, study, and train with his fellow comrades. "If he excelled in judgement and was most courageous in fighting, he was made captain of his company," wrote Plutarch, a Greek historian who wrote a history of Sparta (Kiger, n.d.). He would then be watched and revered by the rest of the boys in his company.

As the boys grew older, they would take part in increasingly brutal competitions of physical prowess. While they had typical foot races and wrestling, like we would have seen in Athens around the same time, there were also contests where two teams would compete to force each other off of an island into the cold, harsh water that awaited. Think of the most brutal boxing match you have ever seen. Even they would have forbidden eye gouging and biting. This was not the case in ancient Sparta. As a matter of fact, Lycurgus—the founder of this brutal system—wrote that the boys and men of the Spartan army would be fed a limited diet. One reason, noted by Xenophon, was that keeping the boys slim would have helped them grow taller. Another, possibly more likely, reason was a matter of practicality. By keeping the boys hungry, it made them more resourceful in finding and gathering food. While stealing was not explicitly encouraged, a Spartan boy who stole food from gardens was more likely to gather resources when he became a soldier. As a matter of fact, although stealing was not encouraged, boys who were caught stealing food were actively punished. Not for the crime of stealing, but for the crime of getting caught (Kiger, n.d.).

Let's take a moment to reflect on all of this. Think deeply about the environment I just described and consider the kind of soldier it could have produced. While not every Spartan man would become a soldier, they were expected to be. As a result, a Spartan warrior trained harshly, was expected to care for himself and his company. They became hard and accustomed to cruel environments. For this reason, the Spartans were considered the best soldiers in all of ancient Greece. If a Spartan man did not become a soldier, he would have been viewed as a failed Spartan and treated as such. However, if he left Sparta and moved to Athens, he would still have a collection of invaluable skills and traits. He would be resourceful, persistent, and observant.

While the Spartans may be an extreme example, there are a few things I want you to take away from them before we move onto the next chapter and start working toward your goals. I keep explaining that HIIT will help you transform in more ways than one, and by giving you a familiar example in the form of the Spartans, I want you to see that you are capable of more than just toning up your body. As I said before, we learn through our environments and the things we take as entertainment can influence us in more ways than just wasting a couple spare hours.

Where Spartan training would be close to 24 hours a day, you only have a half hour with HIIT. As such, you have to make the most of that half hour. By doing this, you will start to feel your body and spirit start to merge together, you will begin to embrace the physical challenges that come your way. Suddenly, taking the stairs instead of the elevator won't seem as difficult as it used to. Instead of taking the bus to a grocery store 10 minutes away, you will find that you have the energy to walk.

There are so many ways to feel good about yourself, and it all started with committing for just a half hour every day and giving it your all!

Chapter 6:

Getting Started With High-Intensity Interval Training

Now that we have covered the history, science, and philosophy of high-intensity interval training, I think it's time we start working toward your goals. In this chapter, I am going to give you some exercises to begin your training. This will include small changes you can make at home, sample workout routines to get your blood flowing, and an introduction to sprinting.

High-intensity interval training is used by track athletes because it conditions their bodies to work quickly and efficiently. My background is in sprinting, and HIIT has been invaluable to me and my personal successes. Sprints, stairs, and hills are the most powerful drills, and if you're able to do it, it's the only exercise you will ever need to do. If it was good enough for the ancient Greeks and Romans, it's good enough for you and me! It's available to everyone of all ages, genders, and abilities. Not to mention, these exercises are used in today's military and have been throughout time. Hill sprints, for example, are used to increase your power and endurance. Both of these are valuable traits to have when you're looking to push and develop beyond your limits.

Before beginning any new training regimen, it's a good idea to consult a medical professional to ensure you don't have any underlying health problems.

The below exercises are amazingly powerful when combined with HIIT. Doing these on a regular basis will rapidly produce transformative results. Please do not confuse rapid with easy. These workouts require you to work out at near maximum, whatever it may be at the time of exercising. If working at your near maximum is too stressful, you start at a lower level of intensity and work your way up. While high intensity is important in HIIT, it's more important that you keep yourself safe and healthy. Once you get the hang of these workouts, you'll be amazed at the rewards you have reaped after such a short amount of time.

Beginner Exercises

Starting any new exercise regimen can be scary and confusing, especially if you don't know where to begin. The purpose of this section is to give you an idea of where to start, how often you should do it, and the results you can expect. I want to start with running and sprinting; as I've mentioned, this is my background. I've felt and seen the benefits, and I would like you to experience them firsthand. When running on flat surfaces, I recommend finding a rubber track—the distances are easier to gauge and if you're up to it, you can use spikes.

Stairs and Hills

A core part of HIIT is the cardiovascular element. There are lots of ways you can incorporate this into your workout. If you are using a workout video on YouTube, the trainer will include something like running in place or jumping jacks.

When you want to design your own workout, you can tailor it to your environment. Start with stairs and hills; use both of these interchangeably before you incorporate sprinting. The below exercise is known as "sprints, stairs, and hills" and is used worldwide by professional athletes. The first thing you want to do is find a hill, and the second thing you want to do is clear it of any debris so that you can avoid injury. A good size for a hill varies according to where you live but try to find one that's at least 30 meters (100 feet) in length. Make sure that the hill is not too steep as it becomes a different workout. This will give you a good range without being too overwhelming.

Start by walking up the hill at a fast pace, taking 30 seconds to a minute, then walk down at a slow, leisurely pace for some active recovery. When you get to the bottom, rest for a minute, then do this again. Repeat at least five times, no more than 10 times if this is one of your first attempts. Keep repeating for as long as you feel able to, each time with a slightly shorter rest. If your hills are short, I recommend doing more reps for maximum gain. As your endurance grows, you can start to incorporate running.

This may not be the way you expected to start HIIT. Don't worry, we are just warming you up. You can still obtain many benefits of HIIT by doing fast walking up hills and stairs with intensity. The objective right now is to get you within the range of exhaustion and push your body. The fitness industry has done an excellent job of convincing you that the only way to get fit and healthy is by going to the gym, having a personal trainer or owning expensive workout equipment. While going to the gym is a great pastime and can provide a motivational environment, you can obtain all the benefits of HIIT at home, in your backyard, or at a local park. The most important thing is that you continue to push yourself from the moment you begin. By its very nature, HIIT encourages you to develop your athletic intuition so you're aware of what you need and are capable of achieving, including if you are able to go faster in any of the exercise. Find that motivation.

Tips for Beginners

When you first start HIIT, you may be tempted to go all out on your first set of reps. I admire your commitment and dedication, but for the sake of your own safety, I encourage you to take it steady. At the start of this book, I talked about personal trainers and workout videos, and how they encourage you to focus on the quality of the rep over the quantity. You are working at maximum intensity in successive blocks of time, so doing 20 bad reps is more likely to cause injury and hold you back while 10 good reps are likely to help you achieve your goals.

With this in mind, you do not have to go all out at the beginning. Instead, with each rep, you should increase the intensity as you increase endurance. This will enhance your ability so you will be able to perform three or more times a week. Ideally, every second day if you choose not to go near your maximum.

As you get stronger and your endurance develops, you can start to incorporate sprinting into your workout. Sprinting is a great way to get your heart rate up at the start of your workout, but you don't have to go for the sprint immediately. Start with light runs to warm up your legs and lungs. Make sure to include dynamic and static stretches.

My advice to you is to be patient and listen to your body. In the beginning stages of high-intensity interval training, your body is getting used to the sudden impact of exercise and influx of oxygen. It will take a few weeks for these changes to fully manifest in your body, so make sure you are performing the exercises correctly.

Finally, as with all forms of exercise, you must ensure that you keep it steady, and get proper rest. We have already explored how HIIT affects our sleep schedules and helps us rest. After a workout, make sure you focus on the quality of sleep you are getting over the quantity. Maintain a regular sleep schedule and keep your body limber and healthy with dynamic and static stretches.

Results

Sprints, stairs, and hills (SSH) is a time-proven form of body conditioning which will enhance your power, strength, and endurance. Spending hours on the treadmill can be a great way to relieve tension, but it won't burn fat or build muscle nearly as fast. Getting out and doing hill and or stair sprints is the choice of countless professional athletes..

Children and teenagers who perform regular SSH conditioning have access to a powerful way of utilizing human growth hormone (HGH) which helps build the body and aids facilitation of brain development, growth, cell regeneration, and cell reproduction. As a result, teenagers benefit from better development. As for adults, you will benefit from general maintenance of health, and gain confidence as you meet your performance goals.

Some other results you can look forward to seeing are the pure power and strength you will feel in everyday life. One of the best ways you can test this is to sprint on flat ground. If you can't find an athletic track near where you live, any flat ground will do. Use these sprints to test your speed. For those of a more scientific mind, I encourage you to set a control experiment and see how well your time improves as a result of sprint training. Start with 50-100 meter sprints, then keep coming back to that control every couple weeks to see how quickly you start smashing your personal best.

Among other things, you can also expect to experience everything else we've discussed in the previous chapters. Increased oxygenation in your brain will lead to more production of brain-derived neurotrophic factors, which will improve the overall health of your brain. Your entire body, on a molecular level, will begin to feel like new. It will take a few weeks for everything to kick in in earnest and once it does, you will be glad you started.

Beginner HIIT Exercises: SPIN and Cycling

Now, I think we should take a look at how HIIT can be applied to a couple of other exercises. Cycling has grown in popularity over the years and so have SPIN classes. If you have either a bike or stationary cycle, you should pay close attention to this section and the same in the next chapter. You can obtain a great number of benefits from implementing a HIIT format into any other exercise.

High-Intensity Interval Cycling

When applied to other exercises, HIIT offers the same base benefits as with sprinting or doing a workout video at home. However, there are differences in your response to the exercise. For example, a sprinter will be able to use the whole body, while cycling you are mostly using your legs. There are muscle group similarities between running and cycling, but they are used in different ways as per the Kriel et al. (2018) study of HIIT when applied to running and cycling. For example running will lengthen legs utilizing a full swing and cycling has a shorter range of motion. For our purposes, we're going to go through a basic set of HIIT, but applied to cycling, which is a very valuable and low-impact form of exercise.

As with any HIIT exercise, you want to push yourself to your near maximum. With cycling, this can be done easier than with running because of the low-impact nature of it, so if running is too hard but you still want to do HIIT, try high-speed cycling, even including intervals up hills. When doing the intervals, push yourself hard for 30 seconds to a minute then cruise and relax for a few minutes then repeat until a state of exhaustion reaches you. Pushing at your near maximum for 30-40 seconds is a challenge when on the road or a mountain due to the dangers involved. My suggestion is to find a smooth quiet street where you live or to do a few circuits around a nearby park before attempting anything more advanced.

Build up your cycling fitness as you feel, the more you do and push further, the easier to increase intensity will be. Cycling on the road is becoming extremely popular and many people reap these benefits. However, it's the longer sessions of constant speed that you may want to avoid. Though it has its place in fitness, we're going after interval sessions in this book. If longer biking sessions are what you desire, then while cruising along, every so often throw in one-minute intervals at near maximum; you will gain so much more. Happy riding.

High-Intensity Interval SPIN

Going to a SPIN class at the gym or simply getting on your stationary cycle at home can be a great source of relief. Trainers use HIIT for a variety of exercise classes regardless of whether they're in-person or online. SPIN is an excellent way to incorporate HIIT into your workout if you do not own a bike or cannot get outside for SSH drills. There are plenty of ways to replicate this on a stationary cycle. Most good cycles will have magnetic resistance as a feature to give you the feeling of being on an incline, and there are plenty of apps and online sessions with professional trainers.

Over the years, there has been a surge in demand for SPIN classes in a variety of forms. While stationary cycles were always available, the rise of Peloton and Echelon has given us wider access to SPIN classes at home. If you don't like sprinting, SPIN can be much more fun. You can find classes and apps which invite you to sing along to the music while you're working out, further stimulating the flow of those all-important endorphins we were talking about earlier. SPIN classes benefit greatly from the Tabata format, and your legs are in constant motion the entire time. Additionally, if you don't feel you are ready to try cycling, SPIN is a great way to introduce you to the sport. It uses the same muscles as cycling, although at a lower intensity. This means you will have to push much harder on a stationary cycle than on a bicycle. You will feel the effects of SPIN stronger than you would with sprinting, and since there is more pressure on your legs as a beginner, you should do a high-intensity interval SPIN session twice a week to begin. Gradually build up to every second day, listening to your body the entire time.

Make use of the magnetic resistance feature on your stationary cycle because this is how you are going to continue to push yourself and become stronger. Your first block should be four or five 30-second rounds at medium intensity, just heavy enough that you can complete a full revolution at a steady, consistent speed. Your second block should feel like you are cycling through thick, heavy mud while still able to complete a full revolution. Be sure to give it your all, and at the same time be careful not to strain or injure yourself.

When you go into the recovery/rest period of your block, set the resistance to zero and just let your legs go free. For your cardio finisher, put the resistance up to just enough so that you can feel it, then go as fast as you can for one minute, repeating once or twice more depending on how you feel. This is a great way to amplify the strength portion of your workout. If you do not feel like doing this alone, joining SPIN classes are recommended, whatever you need to incorporate HIIT.

Chapter 7:

Intermediate and Advanced High-Intensity Interval Training

If you've completed the exercise regimen in the previous chapter, or have already incorporated HIIT for yourself, the transformation has begun. For the next few pages, we're going to introduce flat surface sprinting as the center of your workout. Think about the goal you set a few chapters back. Right now, you're on the path to not only achieving it, but pushing through it and exceeding the expectations you previously set yourself.

The focus here is to enhance the concept of sprints, stairs, and hills conditioning from the previous chapter. At this stage in your training, you're ready to start pushing yourself, and embrace the changes that can only come from high-intensity interval training. Advanced stages of HIIT and sprinting begin to test your limits at full speed thresholds. This is the true key, to run at near or full speed for multiple repetitions. It's very important to note that before you attempt the following exercises, you should be properly stretched and warmed up, otherwise injury is guaranteed. As you continue to train and up your capacity to maximum effort, your transformation will become a reality. Everything you imagined comes to fruition.

Making the Most of Sprints, Stairs, and Hills

At the end of the previous chapter, I advised you to keep an eye on your personal best through a short science experiment. By now, you should have broken your own personal best multiple times and are prepared to begin training on flat surfaces. You've had the first taste of transformation, and now you are ready for the next level.

You can now start sprinting. Start with repetitions between 150-300 meters. If you need to, start at 50 meters and gradually work your way up. Just because it's 50 meter does not mean it's easy: we are talking about near full speed running. The lactic acid comes up quick, so you will want to train through this to develop the speed endurance. This comes with one caveat: the shorter the distance, the more reps you have to do. A longer distance will earn a longer rest, and in both cases you should aim to push yourself to the state of near exhaustion. This is the only way you will be able to go beyond your limits and keep getting stronger. Another great workout I like to add in is to run 150 meters, then rest for maybe 10 seconds, turn around, and run back 50 meters. This mechanism of stacking runs are very powerful and will leave you breathing! (Sample workout stacks: 50/50 - 100/50 - 150/50 - 300/150/50). Mix and match different sprinting lengths and speeds as you see fit; wear spikes if possible, as it is near full speed sprinting, this is the advanced part.

As we move to the next workout day, incorporate hard hills or stair sprinting, alternating between the two every other workout. Alternating between stairs and hills will keep your body guessing and utilize the benefits for those two different training mechanisms. We need to avoid your body getting used to one form of exercise or training, it will start to settle and work less hard. To wrap up, we do sprinting one day, active recovery the next, take another day if you need, then do either hill sprints or stairs, recover, then go back to flat sprints. This way you utilize speed training coupled with strength. Enjoy.

Advanced SPIN and Cycling

Following on from the previous chapter, I would like to continue exploring HIIT applied to SPIN and cycling. Both of these are excellent forms of cardio. While you can't cycle at the gym, you can still learn a lot about the techniques we cover in the cycling sections and apply them to a SPIN bike. In the same way, you might prefer cycling over SPIN, you can still take away some knowledge about resistance and endurance from the SPIN section. Both exercises use the same muscles in different ways and contribute to your metabolism becoming supercharged and your heart rate taking off.

The below exercises are examples of how to improve your speed, cadence and endurance through HIIT. As for every exercise mentioned in this book, you are required to work toward working at near maximum effort for every 30-45 second interval, even taking it to a minute if you feel like it; this is how you maximize your output for the greatest returns. That being said, you should always listen to your body. If you experience pain, stop exercising, and attend to the pain and any injuries that may have developed. Continuing to exercise when you are experiencing pain can turn into a bad injury; however, fatigue is something you can push through to further yourself.

SPIN

I want you to try something a little different. If you've ever been to SoulCycle, have tried Peloton or even just been to a regular SPIN class at the gym, you'll likely know what I'm about to walk you through. On the other hand, for those who have never been to a SPIN class, this entire section is going to sound very weird. More advanced SPIN classes—and techniques in general—incorporate full body movements into the cardio element of exercise. So, a 20-minute SPIN class will deviate far from the normal "go fast, go slow" approach you'll cover in a beginner class. In the comfort of your own home, or even when you're on a stationary cycle at the gym, you can start to incorporate strength training. This is especially beneficial if you want to up your resistance while working out.

As always, begin your HIIT workout by choosing your work:rest ratio. For the purposes of this section, I'm going to use a standard 40:30:30 Tabata formula. If you need help keeping up with the timing, there are countless free "Tabata timer" or "HIIT timer" apps available on your phone. Make sure you also have plenty of water available for your rest breaks and a towel to wipe away any sweat.

I think it's time to start exploring a mix of lower body and upper body when spinning. The idea is pretty novel, and you might think it's pretty funny to lift weights or do resistance training when sitting on a stationary cycle, but it's funny because it's *fun*. Of course, the lower body element is focused on the legs and glutes, while the upper body encourages more movement in the shoulders and arms. Have some resistance ready. Dumbbells will work if you have them, but if you don't then you can use a can of beans or a bottle of water. Anything that gives you some feeling of weight will be helpful in this exercise.

To warm up, start at a relatively quick pace on the stationary bike. Don't add too much resistance yet, just let your legs go free. Then, after about a minute, start adding some resistance. Turn the magnetic resistance up just enough so that you can feel it pushing back against you, then stand up. Be careful here—make sure your feet are completely stable and aren't likely to slip. Stay in this position, and keep going for 40 seconds, then return to your seat and rest for 20 seconds. Repeat as many times as you feel you are able, but I recommend four or five reps to start if you're intermediate. If you're a beginner and want a challenge, go for three or four reps. For the next two blocks of exercise, make sure your legs are comfortable and spinning at a pace you can maintain while still pushing yourself. Your next block of exercise will take you to the upper body. So, after about a minute's rest, take up whatever resistance you have. Staying seated, and continuing to spin, do some dumbbell rows for 30 seconds, then rest for 15 seconds. Repeat up to five times or as many as you feel comfortable doing. For your third and final block, do shoulder presses with your chosen weights for 30 seconds, again repeating up to five times or as many reps as you feel comfortable doing. Once this last block is done, finish off with a 60-second sprint, going as fast as you can. Afterward, cool off with some nice dynamic and static stretches.

Cycling

In the previous chapter, we covered the basics of getting used to cycling out in the open. Now, I want you to start focusing on your technique. For this, you're going to need to get a speedometer and attach it to your bike because I want you to start applying HIIT to your cycling game. There are a lot of things to train when you're cycling which affect not only your health, but your overall safety. These things are cadence and sprinting (which can be done in short bursts). In cycling, cadence is the number of revolutions completed in a single minute of cycling, which will improve as you train more and harder. To help you track this, I recommend using a cadence sensor.

Using the 40:30:30 formula, I want you to train your sprinting muscles. Start off in a light cruise position and in the highest gear that allows you to peddle fast without having to shift; this sprint interval will be for about 45 seconds. For this first set, just go as fast as you are comfortable with. For the next two 30-second sets, however, you need to really up the level of intensity and push yourself to go as fast as you can. Repeat this as many times as you are comfortable doing. The only way to prepare your sprint muscles for sprinting is to actually sprint. When sprinting out in the open, always remain aware of your environment, what's behind, ahead of, or surrounding you—particularly if you are on a road with a lot of heavy traffic. Always take precautions when going out to cycle.

Applying HIIT to Other Exercises

While I'm a proponent of sprint training (as I said, my background is sprinting so I may be a little biased), I recognize that non-sprinters might grow bored of doing SSH drills on a regular basis. Similarly, if you don't own a bicycle or a stationary cycle, you might not feel comfortable investing in one. For this reason, I want you to consider some other exercises where you can apply HIIT to help you make the most of it.

Swimming

If you have any injuries or simply want to take a break from high-impact exercise, you should consider trying high-intensity interval swimming. When you think of swimming, you probably think of a few leisurely laps at your local pool or an Olympic athlete pushing for greatness. In simple terms, high-intensity interval swimming is swimming at or near full speed one length of the pool then resting for a few minutes and repeating until you are done with your workout. Swimming is a very good intense alternative to high impact, and even if you are doing running, adding swimming will be a good addition. It's also a great form of active recovery if you just want to relax with a few leisurely laps, and it can act as a great form of body conditioning for future workouts since it involves so many muscle groups. An all-around good exercise for adding to the HIIT regimen.

Spartan Race Workout Variation

There are also some great workouts you can do from the comfort of your own living room. I mentioned workout videos on YouTube, but there are plenty of programs you can find for free online. This workout I'm going to share with you was modeled after a workout I found from the Spartan Race website. Obstacle course race websites are great places to check out for HIIT workouts because they focus on power and durability, two traits which you absolutely need if you are going to survive something like the Death Race or a Spartan Race (Fetters, n.d.).

For this workout, I recommend finding a local park or, preferably, somewhere sturdy at home, because you are going to be doing a lot of pull-ups. For your cardio element, bring a jump rope or do some jumping jacks. If there are any, use monkey bars for pull-ups. If you're at home, do *not* use a pipe. Use an alternative, such doorway rows or towel pull-ups. For towel pull-ups, make sure that the door opens away from you to reduce risk of injury. Tie overhand knots in the corners of two towels (any towel that's sturdy). Place the knots over the door and close it again making sure that it's secure. One more time for emphasis: make sure that the door opens *away* from you. If you want to do doorway rows, simply stand in front of the door with your feet planted and grab the edges of the doorway. Sit back with your weight on your heels and pull yourself forward.

Choose your pull-up alternative and begin with it. Do it in 45 second bursts, with a 15 second rest before your next set. Your next exercise is a push-up. If you are uncomfortable doing a plank push-up, feel free do go down on your knees. Remember to keep your abdomen parallel to the surface. Go hard for 45 seconds. For your third exercise, you're going to do some squats. If you have a pair of dumbbells or some weight plates lying around, use them, or you can use anything else for resistance if you don't have weights. Squat for 45 seconds, always pushing it to maximum effort. Once the squats are done, take a full minute's recovery and catch your breath, or jog on the spot or do some light jumping jacks if you want to get your heart rate up. If you're still testing the waters with HIIT, repeat this block twice, then finish with a high-intensity cardio finisher of your choice. This is a particularly great set of exercises if you're pressed for time but still want to get some work in. I find that they're best after a stressful day of work. When you think of the buff guy at the gym doing pull-ups, you probably think he's quite aggressive because he's grunting and breathing super hard. Don't worry about him. He's just working off a bad day at the office, and you'll understand his relief once you're done with this workout.

Ashtanga Flow Yoga

Another form of low-impact interval exercise you could try is, surprisingly, ashtanga flow yoga. I keep bringing it up to compare, and there's a good reason for it. Yoga works your body with a healthy level of intensity. Ashtanga relies on consistency between poses and transitions, so you are always moving and flowing like water. Your breathing is guided by the yogi; you are actively encouraged to recognize your limits and work only toward what you are capable of, and the intentions you set at the start of the flow help set up your mind so you can overcome any barriers you face. There are many different styles of yoga, from Vinyasa flow to Dance flow to Mandala flow, and if you want to give them a shot, go ahead. A quick flow can be a great substitute if you don't feel like stretching after SSH drills, and a very good addition to do on recovery days. May you find peace through these yoga exercises.

Further Motivation

Before we finish up and get into the conclusion, I would like to take a few moments to help keep you motivated. The body is an amazing machine. It facilitates its own processes and has its own maintenance systems which keep you up and running. However, all too often we forget that we need to take care of our bodies as well as ourselves. Through a healthy diet and consistent exercise, you can take care of it the way it deserves. We have already explored the incredible ways in which HIIT will benefit your mind, body, and spirit, so we need to take a few moments to really dig deep and explore how to take care of ourselves *after* a workout.

Lactic acid is a biochemical product of anaerobic respiration. After a period of heavy, intense exercise, it starts to build up in your body. The harder and faster you exercise, the more lactic acid will build up in your muscles. Take, for example, running. When you perform several highly intense reps, in a short space of time, lactic acid will build up very quickly. If you do not take measures to release it, it can cause a wide variety of problems, from muscle cramps that last a day to pulled muscles which can take up to a month to heal.

For this reason, after every session of exercise, you need to include a cool down of dynamic and static stretches to help your muscles relax and release. Very valuable tricks to ease and get rid of lactic acid I learned from competitive sprinting is to do ice baths rotated with hot baths. For example, 30 seconds to a minute in waist-deep cold water, then a minute hot. Cycle this about five times or more if needed but finish on cold. This contracting of the muscles will dramatically speed up the healing process. In addition, you can do an Epsom salt bath at home which will further remove toxins from your body. Be sure to finish with stretching after a warm bath; however, be careful not to overstretch in this state.

The next day, your body is going to feel very achy and stiff. It may feel like you don't want to get out of bed, but you need to do a full body stretch. This release of tension is what we're looking for, and although you might not feel up to it, you need to push through the pain in order to make the most of your transformation. The pain you feel the day after is how you know you hit your limit, and by pushing through it with further recovery exercises, you will be able to overcome it even quicker and more efficiently in the future. This is how you push your mind and body that extra step further to excel.

High-intensity interval training pushes you to grow your maximum effort to limits you never would have believed possible. It sounds counterproductive to keep pushing while you are experiencing pain/fatigue, but this is just the first step in developing your athletic intuition. When I was talking about performing that "mental scan" earlier, this is the time for you to put it into practice so you can fully gauge your capacity for your next workout. By training at near maximum effort, you build up your capacity to handle life's difficulties with grace and calm, then you are left wondering if it was even hard at all, a beautiful sense of humor develops.

Committing to this regular level of hard work will shape you in more ways than one. As you get progressively fitter and stronger, your mind will start to change. You'll start to see yourself as a stronger person in all aspects of your life, and you'll have a boost of spirit and self-esteem as never before. Your confidence will explode, you'll start to set clear goals in your life, and you'll start to see home as your place of rest and recovery, a place of relaxation and calm. All of these things are open and available to you as you allow yourself to let go and embrace your transformation. Achieving everything you deserve in life is only the next step.

Conclusion

I strived to provide you during the course of this book plenty of science and philosophy, and I appreciate you for sticking through it with me. It means a lot. When I decided to write this book, it was because I had never seen anyone explore the effects of high-intensity interval training on the mind, body, and spirit in one place. So, rather than you going out and reading three separate books and finding studies on your own, I wanted to concentrate them into one short, digestible book. Now that you have made it this far, I want to use this as an opportunity to revisit all the information in summary.

HIIT and the Human Body

When we covered the effects of HIIT on the human body, you may have probably thought that some of this material is obvious in the fitness world. That being said, I was just as surprised as you when I found out how it affects us on a molecular level. Like you, I had always understood that exercise gave me more energy, but I had never thought to question why. Think back to any cellular anatomy class you had at school, and you probably heard the phrase "the mitochondria are the powerhouse of the cell." When you do regular HIIT, you're stimulating mitochondrial responses, effectively creating more energy for yourself as you go on. By exercising, your mitochondrial responses get stronger, giving you a lot more to work with in the long run and allowing you to consistently achieve your personal best. Nowadays, it seems that everyone and their dog has "the miracle cure" to give you more energy, and it's in the form of a pill or something like that. With high-intensity interval training, you create your own energy by completely organic means.

In addition to the above, HIIT has so many incredible effects on our bodies. Starting with hormone production, HIIT gives your body the chance to work like the incredible machine it is. With the stimulation of human growth hormone (HGH), for instance, your body becomes stronger as a result of better muscle development. However, it's important to note that increased muscle does not necessarily mean increased strength. Instead, you will find your body shape changing as your muscles become better adapted to the increase in intensity of your workouts. Human growth hormone plays such an important role in our bodies, and we often overlook it. When you train efficiently, this powerhouse of a hormone acts as a traffic controller, directing your muscles to cope with the added work effort. You will, as a result, find yourself continually going beyond your personal best and smashing through your limits on a regular basis.

Further, as you perform HIIT exercises, your VO2 max increases, giving you a better basis for body conditioning, which improves your overall well-being. Your heart may feel like it's beating out of your chest half the time, but it gets stronger and healthier as a result of all the exercise you're letting it have. The heart is a muscle and it needs to be worked properly for the best possible functionality; as a result, your blood pressure gets better and so does your heart rate.

Another thing I want to revisit is the effect of HIIT on the base metabolic rate. While exercise in general does affect how many calories we burn, that doesn't mean it significantly affects your base metabolism. You could spend hours on the treadmill, burning all the calories you want in one hour-long chunk, but that doesn't mean your metabolism will continue to burn calories for you. If anything, this could be worse for you since the body gets used to running on a treadmill for a long stretch of time. By pushing your body to its limits with highly intense intervals, you could see your metabolism work up to three times more efficiently, continuing to burn calories for hours—or even days—after a workout. This is due to accelerated thermogenesis, the by-product of calorie burning. By accelerating thermogenesis, you accelerate your metabolism, burning more calories, more effectively.

If you're a parent and want to get your children involved in high-intensity training, go ahead, but it's important to remember that children and adolescents also get burned out. I went over a study which involved 24 adolescent males, and I would also like to revisit this one. Something I want to address, which I think is the most worthwhile aspect of this study, is that the participants saw it as a personal challenge rather than a competition (Abderrahman et al., 2018). While a little friendly competition can be healthy, it can also foster an unhealthy relationship with the ideas of "winning" and "losing." Team sports are a great way to improve strategy and teamwork skills, however this can lead to comparing yourself to other people. When you do HIIT, you only have yourself to compare to. Your personal best is yours alone. As a yogi would say, "your practice is your own. Don't compare yourself with anyone else." We start to see ourselves as an individual person. Working with a team is great, but sometimes we need to be separate, to take a little time to reflect on who we are and who we want to become. This is why I encourage you to set your own goals, set your own path to go down and enjoy the adventure along the way.

HIIT and the Human Mind

Let's take a few moments to recap a few things from the mind and brain sections. Most of the studies we covered might have surprised you with the results. Even though you may have known that exercise is great for the brain, you may not have realized the extent. Increased oxygenation of the brain, for example, and extra stimulation of brain-derived neurotrophic factors are the very source of improved neural functioning. This leads to restructuring of our brain, better memory and stronger decision-making abilities. A lot of people turn to exercise for its physical health benefits, but now that you're armed with information about how much it can help your brain, you can start your HIIT journey knowing that you have a lot to look forward to.

When I introduced a breathing exercise at the start of this book, you probably thought it was a little unconventional. However, as we went on to learn, HIIT is a more mindful exercise than we give it credit for. This is why I chose to start the book with a look at the mind and brain. When we see pictures and videos of personal trainers doing HIIT, they tend to look quite aggressive which can be off-putting, especially if you're new to HIIT. This is why I wanted you to focus on your breath, to give you a gentle nudge into a mindful state and help you prepare to exercise.

The ancient Greeks made sure that their people had a well-rounded education because they believed that the mind, body, and soul were part of the same unit. I couldn't go into full detail about it in this book because the Greek philosophy of exercise is so interesting, it requires its own book. But I will go back to a quote I used earlier: "Lack of activity destroys the good condition of every human being, while movement and methodical physical exercise save and preserve it" (Bray, 2018).

I think Plato had the right idea with this, and we've seen countless examples throughout each section which serve to uphold his statement. In relation to the mind, you start to break down the barriers that were holding you back in life. I spent a lot of focus on the mind because I want you to understand that it doesn't have to be that way. HIIT takes up a half hour every time you do it, and you feel amazing afterward.

We spend so much of our lives focused on work and becoming burned out that we end up not wanting to workout, which leads to poor mental and physical health. When Plato wrote about the benefits of exercise and its relationship with the mind, he was one of the earliest thinkers to establish what we already know: HIIT is good for us. If and when you choose to reread this book, keep Plato's quote in mind.

I do want to briefly revisit the conclusions Van Gelder et al. and Mekari et al. came to, respectively. When the average person mentions that exercise would keep you young, they mean it as a friendly reminder to encourage you to exercise. You may have heard people say it to you when they go on about how they managed to squeeze in a 10-mile run before coming to work. Well, as we saw in the first chapter, exercise really does keep your mind young and healthy. Van Gelder et al. were among the first to show that HIIT can help stave off dementia. This can be seen as a controversial claim, true, since there are so many extraneous factors to consider. However, even if it doesn't, our brains are still active and receive more oxygen, making our neural pathways more functional (Mekari et al., 2020).

I think the mental benefits of HIIT are the most obvious to notice when you start performing these exercises on a regular basis. It can take a while for the body to start to show any signs of changing, but after a couple weeks of getting your blood flowing and your organs pumping, you start to feel less foggy-headed, a lot more clear-minded, and more excited about what the future holds. When I asked you to set your goal, you should pay attention to how you feel mentally at the time of setting it. A lot of athletes keep a journal to record their personal bests; many of them record how they felt before and after exercising. Keeping a journal might seem like an added bit of work when you just want to work out, but if you're interested in tracking your mental health and responses to exercise, this is something I recommend doing. You don't have to write a full dissertation. A simple, "Before working out: I feel nervous," and "After working out: I feel good" will do. Some days you will feel better and other days not so much, so tracking can be an effective tool to measure your progress.

When I brought up the Jung et al. study, it was to illustrate how effective exercise can be for our emotions. Emotional health is a key component of mental health, and it's important that we take the time to enjoy the things in our lives. This study was interesting in particular because it measured affective emotional responses across more types of cardiovascular exercise than just HIIT. With this in mind, it's even more surprising that HIIT was found to be the most enjoyable

(Jung et al., 2014). You might expect steady-state cardio, such as going for a run or a long run on the treadmill to be more enjoyable because it's generally very steady and doesn't require too much effort. My personal theory for this is that HIIT offers us the opportunity to shake things up in our workouts. Humans love variety. The body, mind, and spirit love variety. Varying up our workouts can keep us mentally active, and the short rest breaks in between stop us from dreading the next exercise. When you can get a total body workout in just a half hour every other day, suddenly everything else feels much more attainable.

The Effects of HIIT on the Spirit

With HIIT, you push beyond your limits and consistently outdo yourself. Life is not a competition against anyone apart from yourself. We don't live our lives to compare to others and we can only endeavor to be better than we were yesterday, to enjoy who we are today, and strive to become who we want to be tomorrow. This is something I've learned by doing HIIT coupled with deep meditation. After a workout, you start to reflect on the exercises and everything you accomplished in doing it. Exercise is inherently meditative; we saw that with all the comparisons to yoga and when we explored the ancient Greeks and Spartans. Your athletic intuition develops, which is a part of mindfulness in general. This clarity translates into a healthier mind and better sleep patterns. Your REM sleep cycle improves, allowing you to process things more efficiently as you enter the dream state of sleeping. As a result, you grow spiritually.

I have never seen a book about exercise which dived into the unity of mind, body and spirit, and that's what inspired me to write this. This unity helps us overcome so much. When I talk about the spiritual level of HIIT, I'm talking about the appreciation and development of your non-physical nature beyond the mind and body. We tend to build up a picture of ourselves as a result of what people think of us, and this subconsciously drives our actions. However, this is completely irrelevant. Directly as a result of HIIT, you'll build up a brand new picture of yourself which will supersede all previous versions you created. As you continue to push your boundaries in fitness, you'll find yourself pushing boundaries in all other aspects of your life, growing into an entirely new person.

When I first brought up yoga practice in this book, you were probably wondering what place it held, However, I hope my continued comparison of HIIT to yoga helped you gain some perspective. While these two forms of working out may seem like complete opposites, they serve the same purpose when it comes to spirituality. You may use meditation from yoga in your daily life by just taking a few moments to relax and process your day or you could do a daily flow. Whichever you choose, you've made a conscious choice to set aside some time to breathe and focus on you. Taking a few moments to relax and prepare your body for HIIT by breathing and creating a mindful space can make or break your workout. This develops alongside your athletic intuition, which will continue to surprise you as it unfolds with your growth. When you are consistently pushing your limits in your fitness, you gain an innate understanding of where your limits stand. Once you get used to this, you can start to push yourself even further by crafting entirely new boundaries.

Another thing we explored was the quality of sleep we get as a result of exercise. It doesn't matter how much sleep you get. You could be getting 10+ hours of low-quality sleep a night and still wake up feeling like you barely slept at all. As we saw earlier, HIIT can prepare your brain for a more restful sleep by setting up the REM cycle and stimulating our circadian rhythm. As you go on to perform HIIT exercises, you're going to find that your quality of sleep dramatically improves and full healing takes place. If you're so inclined to do so, I recommend writing down your dreams in the morning. This is a good supplemental exercise to the spiritual benefits you obtain from HIIT, it allows us to explore our subconscious. While a lot will be happening during your transformation as you undergo high-intensity interval training, remember that any development you pursue, it's best to understand it from all angles and reap the spiritual benefits along the way.

Versatility

We have seen just how versatile HIIT can be. I used four of the best-known exercise types to demonstrate it: running, cycling, spinning, and swimming. The key point from this book is that HIIT is simply a way to train, and it's been shown multiple times to be far more effective than steady-state cardio or any trendy new workout regimen which has died out over the years. HIIT has remained relevant despite the odds. It has been used since the days of the ancient Greeks and has experienced a resurgence in popularity as we finally start to appreciate the benefits of it.

You can see in the increased popularity of SPIN and "freestyle combat" classes how HIIT has continued to spread and evolve the way we exercise. There are people who continue with steady-state cardio because it works for them; all they want is a peaceful hour on the treadmill. Some enjoy strength training because it's easier for them to measure their progress. However, there are people—people like you—who have done the steady-state cardio and strength training and decided that they need something else. Something which can be applied to any form of exercise. Whether you want to take a dip in the pool or you want to take a ride out on the country road on your bicycle, you want to challenge yourself. You want to start feeling better and looking better, taking care of your body and your brain in ways you had never previously imagined.

Our brains love variety. I cannot stress that enough. The versatility of HIIT means you have ample opportunities to avoid boredom when exercising. Find workout videos to start with and keep doing them. This way you'll learn what exercises you like, you'll discover how best to push yourself, and you'll start to feel like you can accomplish anything.

Make It Your Own

An important thing that you should take away from this book is that HIIT is available to anyone and everyone. You do not need to go to the gym to do it—it can be done in your living room, kitchen, in the park down the street, and even on your way to or from work. The exercise regimen I suggested in the previous two chapters are guidelines, and I recommend you follow them to get a taste of what your body can accomplish. With that being said, you can vary it up and make this training your own, always trying to work at near maximum capacity. Experiment with the speed of your reps, the distance you want to sprint, the work:rest intervals you choose to train and anything else you can play with. All of this will help you develop your athletic intuition and expand your endurance as your experience with HIIT increases within the first weeks and months of training.

Supplement Your Current Workout

Gyms are a great place to find motivation. In a gym, you are surrounded by people with similar goals and attitudes toward their personal health and well-being. This, in addition to the variety of equipment as well as communal feeling, is why gyms can be such great places to workout. If you enjoy going to the gym and are feeling more than a bit bored or stuck with your current workout regimen, you should consider shaking things up with a course of HIIT at the start or end of your workout. By adding HIIT to the start of your workout, you prepare your body for the hard work to come. This is especially useful for bodybuilders and strength-focused training because it gets the heart rate up, your blood flowing through the body, and excites your muscles. At the end of a workout, it can act as a cardio 'finisher' to amplify all the hard work you've done, and help you break your limits.

As we explored earlier, you can employ HIIT into a wide variety of workouts. Everything from spinning to swimming can be covered. You may remember swimming lessons or gym class as a child, where you had to run at maximum speed for what felt like forever but was in reality about 30 or so seconds. When you apply this to your workout as an adult, you start to appreciate the improvements you are capable of making.

What Works For You

What works for some might not work for others. Working out in a gym environment, you will see a wide variety of training happening at once from a powerlifter setting a new personal best, to a sprinter using the stair climber. Outside of the gym, you'll probably see people doing yoga in the summertime and people running half-marathon distances in the spring as they get ready for events. You might even come across more people doing HIIT as you start to get more serious about your personal transformation. All of these are great workout options, but do not feel tempted to copy everyone you see. That powerlifter probably has a couple years of training under their belt, and the half-marathon runner had to gradually build up their endurance for months. If you're just starting with HIIT, you have to do what works for you. The sprints, stairs, and hills training I walked you through in a previous chapter is a way of conditioning your body to get used to something new and intense, use it, it has worked for me through many years. If you find that it doesn't work for you, then I fully encourage you to find something that does work. That could be doing a daily HIIT video on YouTube every morning, a quick Vinyasa flow in the evening, or just going out for an interval-based run after lunch. Just don't forget to push. This is the key component to HIIT—constantly push yourself to reach your maximum potential. This potential expands and grows as you push your boundaries and endurance thresholds, you'll be able to achieve three-fold transformation in the body, mind, and spirit through high-intensity interval training. May it work for you.

Explore

"The journey not the arrival matters" — T.S. Eliot (Goodreads, n.d.).

You have before you the beginnings of an amazing opportunity to explore this transformation within yourself, your entire being, physically, mentally and spiritually, monitor its progress and expand on it, and always continue to believe and trust in yourself. Realize that high-intensity interval training will be as hard as you make it, so make sure it counts, in the end it will be extremely rewarding. Use this to your advantage. May you achieve what you desire for yourself and the goals you set, and may the world open up to you the eventualities you seek.

Author's Note

Dear Reader,

Thank you for purchasing my book and taking the time to read through the material. I hope you received as much enjoyment from it as I did writing it. May you take from it a new sense of direction and purpose toward striving for your own personal growth.

I would like to take this time to humbly ask that you leave for me an honest review on whatever platform you purchased this book from, as I do take the time to read all of them to further assist me in my growth and to make improvements to my published works. This would be greatly appreciated. I offer you my sincerest gratitude in taking the time to leave a review for me.

May we all achieve our fullest potential and then push even further.

And so it is.

Most Gratefully Written,

Paul

References

A Misunderstanding Of High Intensity Interval Training. (2017, November 17). Science of Running. https://www.scienceofrunning.com/2017/11/a-misunderstanding-of-high-intensity-interval-training.html?v=47e5dceea252

Abderrahman, A. B., Rhibi, F., Ouerghi, N., Hackney, A. C., Saeidi, A., & Zouhal, H. (2018). Effects of Recovery Mode during High Intensity Interval Training on Glucoregulatory Hormones and Glucose Metabolism in Response to Maximal Exercise. *Journal of athletic enhancement, 7*(3), 292. https://doi.org/10.4172/2324-9080.1000292

Asghar, R. (n.d.). *HIIT For The Mind: 15 Minutes To Supercharge Your Workday.* Forbes. Retrieved February 20, 2021, from https://www.forbes.com/sites/robasghar/2020/06/09/hiit-for-the-mind-15-minutes-to-supercharge-your-workday/?sh=353bf0902b8d

Astorino, T. A., Allen, R. P., Roberson, D. W., & Jurancich, M. (2012). Effect of High-Intensity Interval Training on Cardiovascular Function,

&OV0312;o2max, and Muscular Force. *Journal of Strength and Conditioning Research*, *26*(1), 138–145. https://doi.org/10.1519/jsc.0b013e318218dd77

Astorino, Todd & Schubert, Matt. (2018). Changes in fat oxidation in response to various regimes of high intensity interval training (HIIT). European Journal of Applied Physiology. 118. 10.1007/s00421-017-3756-0.

Batacan, R. B., Duncan, M. J., Dalbo, V. J., Tucker, P. S., & Fenning, A. S. (2016). Effects of high-intensity interval training on cardiometabolic health: a systematic review and meta-analysis of intervention studies. *British Journal of Sports Medicine*, *51*(6), 494–503. https://doi.org/10.1136/bjsports-2015-095841

Bray, E. (2018, November 28). *Plato On Exercise*. Ernie Bray. https://www.erniebray.com/blog/2018/11/25/plato-on-exercise.

Britanniae, B. (2017, January 18). *Fitness in Ancient Rome*. Latin Language Blog | Language and Culture of the Ancient Latin-Speaking World. https://blogs.transparent.com/latin/fitness-in-ancient-rome/

Brown, E. (n.d.). *Ancient Greek Athletic Training*. LIVESTRONG.COM.

https://www.livestrong.com/article/349071-ancient-greek-athletic-training/

Cahn, B. R., Goodman, M. S., Peterson, C. T., Maturi, R., & Mills, P. J. (2017). Yoga, Meditation and Mind-Body Health: Increased BDNF, Cortisol Awakening Response, and Altered Inflammatory Marker Expression after a 3-Month Yoga and Meditation Retreat. *Frontiers in Human Neuroscience*, *11*. https://doi.org/10.3389/fnhum.2017.00315

Cell Press. (2017, March 7). How exercise -- interval training in particular -- helps your mitochondria stave off old age. *ScienceDaily*. Retrieved March 1, 2021 from www.sciencedaily.com/releases/2017/03/170307155214.htmEnright, Stephanie & Unnithan, Viswanath & Heward, Clare & Withnall, Louise & Davies, David. (2006). Effect of High-Intensity Inspiratory Muscle Training on Lung Volumes, Diaphragm Thickness, and Exercise Capacity in Subjects Who Are Healthy. Physical therapy. 86. 345-54. 10.1093/ptj/86.3.345.

Copeland, J. L., Consitt, L. A., & Tremblay, M. S. (2002). Hormonal Responses to Endurance and Resistance Exercise in Females Aged 19-69 Years. *The Journals of Gerontology Series A: Biological Sciences and Medical Sciences*, *57*(4), B158–B165. https://doi.org/10.1093/gerona/57.4.b158

Di Blasio, Andrea & Izzicupo, Pascal & Tacconi, Laura & Santo, Serena & Leogrande, Marina & Bucci, Ines & Ripari, Patrizio & Baldassarre, Angela & Napolitano, Grazia. (2014). Acute and delayed effects of high-intensity interval resistance training organization on cortisol and testosterone production. The Journal of sports medicine and physical fitness. 56.

Effect of High-Intensity Inspiratory Muscle Training on Lung Volumes, Diaphragm Thickness, and Exercise Capacity in Subjects Who Are Healthy. (2006). *Physical Therapy*. https://doi.org/10.1093/ptj/86.3.345

Engel, F., Härtel, S., Strahler, J., Wagner, M. O., Bös, K., & Sperlich, B. (2014). Hormonal, Metabolic, and Cardiorespiratory Responses of Young and Adult Athletes to a Single Session of High-Intensity Cycle Exercise. *Pediatric Exercise Science*, *26*(4), 485–494. https://doi.org/10.1123/pes.2013-0152

Europe PMC. (2019). *Europe PMC*. Europepmc.org. https://europepmc.org/article/med/32301856

Fetters, A.K. (n.d.). *Tight for Time? Do This QUICK HIIT Workout to Build Power and De-Stress*. Spartan Race. Retrieved February 24, 2021, from https://www.spartan.com/blogs/unbreakable-training/quick-hiit-workout

Goodreads. (n.d.). A quote by T.S. Eliot. Retrieved March 05, 2021, from https://www.goodreads.com/quotes/657162-the-journey-not-the-arrival-matters

HIIT Swim Workout to Incinerate Fat | Shape Plus. (2017, December 13). ShapePlus. https://www.shapeplus.com/hiit-swim-workout-to-incinerate-fat/

How exercise -- interval training in particular -- helps your mitochondria stave off old age. (n.d.). ScienceDaily. https://www.sciencedaily.com/releases/2017/03/170307155214.htm

Hötting, K., & Röder, B. (2013). Beneficial effects of physical exercise on neuroplasticity and cognition. *Neuroscience and Biobehavioral Reviews*, *37*(9 Pt B), 2243–2257. https://doi.org/10.1016/j.neubiorev.2013.04.005

Jamie, P. (2016, January 1). *Physiological responses to concurrent resistance exercise and high-intensity interval training: implications for muscle hypertrophy.* https://repository.lboro.ac.uk/articles/thesis/Physiological_responses_to_concurrent_resistance_exercise_and_high-intensity_interval_training_implications_for_muscle_hypertrophy/9608852

Jung, M. E., Bourne, J. E., & Little, J. P. (2014). Where does HIT fit? An examination of the affective response to high-intensity intervals in comparison to continuous moderate-and continuous vigorous-intensity exercise in the exercise intensity-affect continuum. *PloS one*, *9*(12), e114541.

Kiger, P. J. (n.d.). *How Sparta Used Harsh Training to Produce "Perfect" Warriors.* HISTORY. https://www.history.com/news/sparta-warriors-training

Kong, Z., Sun, S., Liu, M., & Shi, Q. (2016). Short-Term High-Intensity Interval Training on Body Composition and Blood Glucose in Overweight and Obese Young Women. *Journal of diabetes research*, *2016*, 4073618. https://doi.org/10.1155/2016/4073618

Korman, N., Armour, M., Chapman, J., Rosenbaum, S., Kisely, S., Suetani, S., Firth, J., & Siskind, D. (2019). High Intensity Interval Training (HIIT) for people with Severe Mental Illness: A systematic review & meta-analysis of intervention studies– considering diverse approaches for mental and physical recovery. *Psychiatry Research*, 112601. https://doi.org/10.1016/j.psychres.2019.112601

Kriel, Yuri & Askew, Christopher & Solomon, Colin. (2018). The effect of running versus cycling high-intensity intermittent exercise on local tissue oxygenation and perceived enjoyment in 18–30-year-old sedentary men. PeerJ. 6. e5026. 10.7717/peerj.5026.

Laursen, P. B., & Jenkins, D. G. (2002). The Scientific Basis for High-Intensity Interval Training. *Sports Medicine*, *32*(1), 53–73. https://doi.org/10.2165/00007256-200232010-00003

Machado, Alexandre & Baker, Julien & Nunes, Rodolfo & Vale, Rodrigo & Figueira junior, Aylton & Bocalini, Danilo. (2017). Body Weight based in high intensity interval training: the new calisthenics ?. Manual Therapy, Postutology & Rehabilitation Journal. 15. 10.17784/mtprehabjournal.2017.15.448.

Malik, A. A., Williams, C. A., Weston, K. L., & Barker, A. R. (2019). Perceptual and Cardiorespiratory Responses to High-Intensity Interval Exercise in Adolescents: Does Work Intensity Matter? *Journal of Sports Science & Medicine*, *18*(1), 1–12. https://pubmed.ncbi.nlm.nih.gov/30787646/

Martland, R. (2020, May). *T147. CAN HIGH INTENSITY INTERVAL TRAINING (HIIT) IMPROVE PHYSICAL AND MENTAL HEALTH OUTCOMES? A META-REVIEW OF THE GLOBAL BENEFITS OF HIIT AND FOCUSED SYSTEMATIC REVIEW OF THE*

EFFECTS OF HIIT IN MENTAL DISORDERS.
https://www.researchgate.net/publication/3414
84815_T147_CAN_HIGH_INTENSITY_INT
ERVAL_TRAINING_HIIT_IMPROVE_PHY
SICAL_AND_MENTAL_HEALTH_OUTCO
MES_A_META-
REVIEW_OF_THE_GLOBAL_BENEFITS_
OF_HIIT_AND_FOCUSED_SYSTEMATIC_
REVIEW_OF_THE_EFFECTS_OF_HIIT_IN
_MENTAL_D

Martínez-Díaz, I. C., Escobar-Muñoz, M. C., & Carrasco, L. (2020). Acute Effects of High-Intensity Interval Training on Brain-Derived Neurotrophic Factor, Cortisol and Working Memory in Physical Education College Students. *International journal of environmental research and public health*, *17*(21), 8216. https://doi.org/10.3390/ijerph17218216

Mekari, S., Earle, M., Martins, R., Drisdelle, S., Killen, M., Bouffard-Levasseur, V., & Dupuy, O. (2020). Effect of High Intensity Interval Training Compared to Continuous Training on Cognitive Performance in Young Healthy Adults: A Pilot Study. *Brain Sciences*, *10*(2), 81. https://doi.org/10.3390/brainsci10020081

Mellow, M. L., Goldsworthy, M. R., Coussens, S., & Smith, A. E. (2020). Acute aerobic exercise and neuroplasticity of the motor cortex: A systematic review. *Journal of Science and Medicine in Sport*, *23*(4), 408–414. https://doi.org/10.1016/j.jsams.2019.10.015

Peake, J. M., Tan, S. J., Markworth, J. F., Broadbent, J. A., Skinner, T. L., & Cameron-Smith, D. (2014). Metabolic and hormonal responses to isoenergetic high-intensity interval exercise and continuous moderate-intensity exercise. *American Journal of Physiology-Endocrinology and Metabolism*, *307*(7), E539–E552. https://doi.org/10.1152/ajpendo.00276.2014

Petrofsky, J., Laymon, M., Altenbernt, L., Gonzales, K., & Guinto, C. (2011). Post Exercise Basal Metabolic Rate Following a 6 Minute High Intensity Interval Workout. *The Journal of Applied Research* •, *11*(2). https://jrnlappliedresearch.com/articles/Vol11I ss2/Petrofsky1.pdf

The Rugby Republic. (2016, March 28). Sauna, recovery and hgh! http://www.therugbyrepublic.com/performance /2016/3/28/sauna-recovery-and-hgh#:~:text=The%20heat%20from%20a%20sa una,those%20to%20the%20various%20tissues.& amp;text=It%20is%20also%20suggested%20that ,minute%20session%20straight%20vs%20breaks .

Stokes, Keith & Nevill, Mary & Cherry, Paul & Lakomy, Henryk & Hall, George. (2004). Effect of 6 weeks of sprint training on growth hormone responses to sprinting. European journal of applied physiology. 92. 26-32. 10.1007/s00421-003-1038-5.

Vella, C. A., Taylor, K., & Drummer, D. (2017). High-intensity interval and moderate-intensity continuous training elicit similar enjoyment and adherence levels in overweight and obese adults. *European Journal of Sport Science*, *17*(9), 1203–1211. https://doi.org/10.1080/17461391.2017.1359679

Walker, M. (2019, October 8). *Emile Coue method and 4 Unusual Suggestions - CBT*. https://www.cbtcognitivebehavioraltherapy.com/emile-coue-method/

Yeager, S. (2018, November 29). *The Ultimate Guide to High-Intensity Interval Training for Runners*. Runner's World; Runner's World. https://www.runnersworld.com/training/a25335864/high-intensity-interval-training/

Zhang, Haifeng & Tong, Tomas & Qiu, Weifeng & Zhang, Xu & Zhou, Shi & Liu, Yang & He, Yuxiu. (2017). Comparable Effects of High-Intensity Interval Training and Prolonged Continuous Exercise Training on Abdominal Visceral Fat Reduction in Obese Young Women.

Journal of Diabetes Research. 2017. 1-9. 10.1155/2017/5071740.

Zurita-Ortega, F., Chacón-Cuberos, R., Cofre-Bolados, C., Knox, E., & Muros, J. J. (2019). Correction: Relationship of resilience, anxiety and injuries in footballers: Structural equations analysis. *Plos one*, *14*(2), e0212083.

Made in United States
Orlando, FL
23 September 2024